Introduction to Robotics in Minimally Invasive Neurosurgery

Mohammed Maan Al-Salihi
R. Shane Tubbs · Ali Ayyad
Tetsuya Goto · Mohammad Maarouf
Editors

Introduction to Robotics in Minimally Invasive Neurosurgery

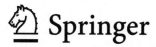 Springer

Editors
Mohammed Maan Al-Salihi
College of Medicine
University of Baghdad
Baghdad, Iraq

Ali Ayyad
Department of Neurosurgery
Hamad General Hospital
Doha, Qatar

Mohammad Maarouf
Department of Neurosurgery
Stereotactic and Functional
Neurosurgery, Beta Clinic Bonn
Bonn, Germany

R. Shane Tubbs
Department of Neurosurgery
Tulane University
New Orleans, LA
USA

Tetsuya Goto
Department of Neurosurgery
St. Marianna University School of Medicine
Kawasaki, Kanagawa
Japan

ISBN 978-3-030-90864-5   ISBN 978-3-030-90862-1   (eBook)
https://doi.org/10.1007/978-3-030-90862-1

This Springer imprint is published by the registered company Springer Nature Switzerland AG
The registered company address is: Gewerbestrasse 11, 6330 Cham, Switzerland

*This book is dedicated to my beloved parents, brothers, and sisters.
And to my wife Yaman and my children Abdulrahman and Sarrah Hanan in acknowledgment of their understanding and support.*

Mohammad Maarouf

Foreword

Pioneers in surgery—like early explorers who sought goals like the North Pole, the South Pole, the top of Mt. Everest—are sometimes ill-fated. The inventor of one of the first surgical robots—ROBODOC for precision CT-guided femur reaming in hip replacement—is an example. Howard A. Paul, a forward-looking veterinarian at the University of California, Davis (California, USA)—who was affectionately called by his initials "HAP"—sadly succumbed to leukemia in 1993 at the age of 44. I was fortunate in the 1990s to visit the manufacturing facilities for ROBODOC (and NeuroMate) in Lyon (France), and also to participate in another building block of neurosurgical robotics: the innovative program for image-guided surgery at Vanderbilt University. Fortunately, Hap Paul lives on in the annual "Hap Paul Award" of the International Society for Technology in Arthroplasty.

The editors of *Introduction to Robotics in Minimally Invasive Neurosurgery* are pioneers in their own right—particularly the lead editor, Mohammed Maan Al-Salihi. To assemble such an informative book on cutting-edge neurosurgery while working in one of the world's political "hot spots" requires dedication and insight far above the norm.

"*IRMIN*" is remarkable in several ways:

- It comprehensively reviews the field from both the anatomical aspect (vascular, spine) and the technological aspect (stereotactic, endoscopic).
- It covers the timeline from its beginnings in the 1980s (and groundwork laid decades earlier) to the future of neurosurgical robotics (artificial intelligence (AI), internet of things (IoT), brain-to-brain interface (BTBI)).
- Each chapter can be read "stand-alone." Although this results in some overlap and repetition, the reader can quickly access the specific information desired.
- The documentation is exemplary. Most chapters have dozens of references, up-to-date and relevant; one chapter has 147 references!

By tackling neurosurgical robotics, Dr. Al-Salihi and colleagues have addressed the area that is destined to be the core of neurosurgery in the second half of the twenty-first century (if not before then!). No doubt a second edition will document progress in various aspects:

- Minimally invasive access to the nervous system will undoubtedly progress. As Rodolfo Llinas (Emeritus Chair of Neurophysiology at New York University) envisaged in 2005, one can drive the endovascular pathways not only along the "superhighways" of the internal carotid and other large arteries for coiling and stenting but also along the "alleyways" of the capillaries that reach every nook and cranny of the nervous system. He showed one can record and stimulate the nervous system utilizing electrodes within the blood vessels. And, as suggested by Kendall Lee at the Mayo Clinic, one can poke a micron-size catheter through the capillary wall to investigate (and manipulate!) the brain parenchyma—red blood cells are ten times the diameter of the penetrating catheter and thus will not leak out.
- Neuroprostheses will evolve to replace parts for nervous systems defects. Researchers in Italy, the Netherlands, and the USA have developed a prototype bioinspired artificial synapse. Being able to replace defective neurons, nerve fibers, and synapses—either with artificial prostheses or stem-cell derived replacements—will revolutionize the treatment of nervous system disorders.
- The brain-cloud interface (B/CI) and brain-to-brain interface (BTBI) will take neurosurgical robotics into the realm of neurosurgical "crowdsourcing." A group at the University of Washington in Seattle, WA, USA, has shown that one person being monitored by EEG can—through the internet and transcranial magnetic stimulation—remotely control the motor function of another person. In essence, the second person becomes a slave of the first.

The implications of advanced B/CI and BTBI are of concern, as the example above illustrates. As the tools for neurosurgical robotics become more sophisticated, the ethical aspects will need to be addressed. Psychosurgery has repeatedly been accused of overstepping the boundaries of medical ethics; neurosurgical robotics should avoid this fate.

Seventy-five years ago, Norbert Wiener—considered the "Father of Cybernetics" (cybernetics—including feedback guidance—being a cornerstone of neurosurgical robotics)—was confronted with a similar dilemma. He denied a request from a company for a report on guided missiles he authored during World War II, arguing in a letter that appeared in both the *Atlantic Monthly* and the *Bulletin of Atomic Scientists*:

> ...in any investigation of this kind the scientist ends by putting unlimited powers in the hands of the people whom he is least inclined to trust with their use.

Let us hope, by creating next-generation neurosurgical robotics, that we are not unleashing unlimited powers for "mind control" by the people we are least inclined to trust with their use.

As Lars Leksell, inventor of stereotactic radiosurgery, observed:

> A fool with a tool is still a fool.

By surveying neurosurgical robotics so comprehensively, Dr. Al-Salihi and colleagues have laid the groundwork necessary to avoid neurosurgical robotics becoming at best a "fool's errand" and at worst—in the hands of inhumane fools—a tool for exploitation of the human mind.

June, 2021

Russell J. Andrews
Nanotechnology and Smart Systems
NASA Ames Research Center,
Moffett Field, CA, USA

Foreword

I have read with great satisfaction the book *Introduction to Robotics in Minimally Invasive Neurosurgery* by the editors Dr. Mohammed Maan Al-Salihi, MD, R. Shane Tubbs, MD, Ali Ayyad, MD, Tetsuya Goto, MD, and Mohammad Maarouf, MD.

Although Robotics began to be applied to medicine several decades ago, we can say that this area of modern neurosurgery is like a child who is just taking his first steps and that probably, in a not too distant time, will amaze us with the applications that we will find for it and the usefulness it will have for modern medicine and neurosurgery. The fantasy of humankind finally replaced by machines, by a "robot," has ceased to frighten the scientist, gradually giving way to the concept of robotics complementing and perfecting his task. It is necessary to read this book so that we can keep in mind when in the future we will see minimally invasive neurosurgical techniques assisted by robotics. The main value of this fascinating work is not in the details or the learning of a surgical technique, but in the fact that the reader can visualize and explore the various paths in which this child, who is Robotic Neurosurgery, is already taking a leading role in major neurosurgical centers in the world. This book is helpful in understanding where we are going in neurosurgery and robotics.

The different chapters are practical; the most important concepts are clearly explained and quickly provide the reader with the necessary knowledge to imagine how much robotic technology can improve our surgical interventions in different areas such as spinal, vascular, endoscopic neurosurgery, among others.

I believe that just as the surgical microscope first and then computers and images gained a place in neurosurgery operating rooms, robotics will be another important tool in the near future that is here to stay.

I also want to emphasize that it caused me great satisfaction to receive and preface this work when I saw that its leading editor comes from one of the places on the planet that has suffered the most in many years, Iraq—a country that endured difficulties and adversities of all kinds and yet it is capable of giving medical professionals like Dr. Mohammed Maan Al-Salihi, MD, and other authors, who wrote a book about medicine practically of the future. This is really exciting. I want to congratulate you for the work done on this book. Furthermore, I want to tell you that it has been an honor for me to write this foreword, and I also want to recommend your book mainly for young neurosurgeons who want to explore robotics applied to minimally invasive neurosurgery as a specialty to follow.

Finally, I want to tell you that a country whose young doctors choose the path of science and innovation, ethics, merit, and knowledge is a country that undoubtedly has ahead not only great professionals but also a bright future.

Roberto R. Herrera
Neurosurgical Department and Intraoperative MRI
Belgrano Adventist Clinic,
Buenos Aires, Argentina

Foreword

Robotics will definitely bring us a new horizon of Neurosurgery.

What do we expect Robotics and AI to bring us? The utmost goals for such systems are the ability to treat challenging lesions safely and securely, especially ACCURACY and DEXTERITY beyond human skills and knowledge. At the same time, safety, accuracy, durability, versatility, and cost-benefits are the realistic requirements for the system to be efficiently developed and distributed.

For that purpose, various imaging techniques, computer technology, and robotic systems have been developed. The book *Introduction to Robotics in Minimally Invasive Neurosurgery* by Dr. Al-Salihi MM, et al. nicely summarizes the current technology and future goals of robotic surgery in the field of neurosurgery. AI which I prefer to read "Augmented Intelligence" rather than "Artificial Intelligence" is also an essential part of our future operative theater. Advanced virtual reality, augmented intelligence, and robotics will be assisting us greatly, not replacing us in the OR in the 2030s.

The Alchemi could not yield GOLD, but it brought us vast knowledge in Chemistry.

Robotic technology does not only advance our skills but also provides clues on how to digitalize surgical procedures and understand the science behind the surgical techniques.

To guide appropriate developments and applications of such technology, we should be involved in the essential processes of the development. We should never be driven by market-oriented forces, or use robotics just for the interests. We need to know the limits and yet use the benefits of such technology. Otherwise, robotic surgery will follow the route and history of Alchemi.

Hope this book will guide you.

KNOW the ROBOTICS' BENEFITS and LIMITS.

Akio Morita
Dean, Graduate School of Medicine
and Professor and Chairman
Department of Neurological Surgery, Nippon Medical School
Tokyo, Japan

President, Japanese Society for Skull Base Surgery
Osaka, Japan

Secretary, World Federation of Neurological Societies
Nyon, Switzerland

Foreword

"The glory of medicine is that it is constantly moving forward, that there is always more to learn." This quote, stated by a pioneer of the twentieth century, Dr. William J. Mayo, not only denotes passion and dedication for our field, but also envisions and inspires us towards innovation and the search for greatness. *Introduction to Robotics in Minimally Invasive Neurosurgery* is the first edition of an excellent book that explores and presents an overview of technological advances poised to help the medical practice. Dr. Mohammed Maan Al-Salihi gathered a group of experts in the surgical, neurological, and engineering fields to guide us through this aspect of neurosurgery, which includes, but is not limited to, surgical procedures, augmented reality, supporting systems, and artificial intelligence. This text expands our understanding of current and future robotic technologies used in the surgical treatment of central nervous system diseases and encourages neurosurgeons to embrace innovative tools that push the boundaries of traditional practice.

The authors describe present and upcoming applications of robots in neurosurgery. The book concisely covers the broad topics involved with diagnostic and surgical protocols, guided procedures, image processing, robotic assistance, geometrical accuracy, and automation. The unique interaction between robotics and minimally invasive procedures in neurosurgery is detailed while exploring specific nuances and challenges of stereotactic, endovascular, endoscopic, and spinal techniques. From assisted aneurysm coiling, stent deployment, and brain biopsy, to precise pedicle screw placement, the role of robotics in surgery is well outlined.

We live in an unparalleled time when science and technology interact and move us forward. The editors have taken the challenge of organizing this topic in a meaningful approach, which will provide the neurosurgeon with a trustworthy source of information.

This book will be important for our field, and it will help us attain the "two objects of medical education: to heal the sick and to advance the science" (Charles H. Mayo).

Fidel Valero-Moreno
Neurologic Surgery
Mayo Clinic Florida,
Jacksonville, FL, USA

Alfredo Quiñones-Hinojosa
William J. and Charles H. Mayo,
Neurologic Surgery
Mayo Clinic Florida
Jacksonville, FL, USA

Foreword

The word "robot" conjures up a variety of images, from human-like machines that exist to serve their creators to the Rover Sojourner, which explored the Martian landscape as part of the Mars Pathfinder mission. Some people may alternatively perceive robots as dangerous technological ventures that will someday lead to the demise of the human race, either by outsmarting us and taking over the world or by turning us into completely technology-dependent beings who passively sit by and program robots to do all of our work.

So, what exactly is a robot? Several definitions exist, the Robot Institute of America defined it in 1979 as "a reprogrammable, multifunctional manipulator designed to move material, parts, tools, or specialized devices through various programmed motions for the performance of a variety of task." While in Webster's Dictionary it is defined as "an automatic device that performs functions normally ascribed to humans or a machine in the form of a human."

The idea of an industrial robot was born from American engineer George Charles Devol Jr. in 1954. He later on met Joseph Frederick Engelberger, an entrepreneur and the man who would come to be known as "the father of robotics" and convinced him of the potential of his idea. In 1961, they founded Unimation Inc. In the following year, they succeeded in the trial production of the world's first industrial robot, the Unimate. General Motors Company showed interest in the Unimate, and with the deployment of the robot in the GM's die-casting factory, the world's first industrial robot was brought to life and the practical use of industrial robots commenced in 1962. Since then, industrial robots have transformed not only the manufacturing industry but many more parts of industry and even our daily life.

Academia also made much progress in the creation of new robots. In 1958 at the Stanford Research Institute, a research team developed a robot called "Shakey." Shakey was far more advanced than the original Unimate, which was designed for specialized, industrial applications. Shakey could wheel around the room, observe the scene with his television "eyes," move across unfamiliar surroundings, and to a certain degree, respond to his environment. He was given his name because of his wobbly and clattering movements.

But it took nearly three decades before robotic technology entered the surgical industry, beginning with applications to improve accuracy and precision in neurosurgery during stereotactic brain biopsies and in the field of orthopedics for joint alignment. The first documented use of a robot-assisted surgical procedure occurred in 1985 when the PUMA 560 robotic surgical arm was used in a neurosurgical biopsy! The first laparoscopic procedure involving a robotic system, a cholecystectomy, was performed in 1987. The following year the same PUMA system was used to perform a robotic transurethral resection. In 1990 the AESOP system produced by Computer Motion became the first system approved by the Food and Drug Administration (FDA) for its endoscopic surgical procedure. In that period there were great expectations for robotic neurosurgery because it would allow for greater precision when used in minimally invasive surgeries. But the progress was first outside the neurosurgical field. In 2000, the da Vinci Surgery System broke new ground by becoming the first robotic surgery system approved by the FDA for general laparoscopic surgery. This was the first time the FDA approved an all-encompassing system of surgical instruments, scopes, and camera utensils. Since then, robotic assistance emerged as a tool to overcome problematic ergonomics limiting dexterity and the pitfalls of bidimensional imaging associated with traditional endoscopic approaches, with roles quickly expanding to urologic, gastrointestinal, cardiac, maxillofacial, ophthalmologic, and gynecologic procedures.

Although neurosurgical history is intricately linked to the predecessors of today's robot platforms, neurosurgery has not seen as broad an adoption of robotic techniques as it was expected in the 1990s, despite the rich history of technical neurosurgical innovation, e.g., in stereotaxy, in functional neurosurgery and neuronavigation. And also, despite the fact that many aspects of neurosurgery lend themselves perfectly to the need and implementation of robotics. I think that the reason why robotic neurosurgery has been slow in its development has not been for lack of creativity or desire, but rather because of the inherent complexity of microneurosurgical operations, even more so of minimally invasive and endoscopic procedures. It will be impossible to have just one robot that has all the competencies to fulfill such specific needs as, e.g., endoscopic removal of a ventricular tumor or placing pedicle screws in multilevel spinal fusion.

With this *Introduction to Robotics in Minimally Invasive Neurosurgery*, the editorial team of Mohammed Maan Al-Salihi succeeded in a comprehensive academic compilation of the current status of robotic surgery in many aspects of contemporary neurosurgery. Chapters in the book are primarily written by experts in their respective fields, with excellent overviews of the use of robotics in vascular neurosurgery, stereotactic neurosurgery, and, most extensively, in neuroendoscopy. But it also includes areas like artificial intelligence, internet of things, use of robots in training of neurosurgeons and even nanorobotics. For everyone who is interested in this field and wants to know where the field stands right now, this is a "must-read."

J. André Grotenhuis,
Radboud University Nijmegen Medical Center
Nijmegen, The Netherlands

Preface

Surgery is a very old art that has evolved since prehistoric times. Although certainly practiced earlier, the first documented surgical text is the Edwin Smith papyrus which was written sometimes after 1700 BC (Goodrich 2004). Surgery and its nuances are discussed along with case examples including injuries to the cranium and spine. The modern operating room would be bewildering to the surgeon of centuries past. Today, technology is used almost reflexively in the modern operating theater. Recent advances that are used by the modern surgeon include various computerized technologies such as intraoperative virtual reality and image guidance modalities. Neurosurgeons have also embraced these latest advances. These include the above noted entities and various electronic monitoring systems, improved applications of the surgical microscope such as imaging overlay and ability to see injected fluorescent dyes in order to better identify pathological tissues. Hands-free vision enhancing devices that offer an alternative to the surgical microscope are also now available.

Probably the most technologically advanced device being used in modern neurosurgery and the focus of the present textbook is robotics. Although such devices have been used in other surgical specialties for a longer period of time, e.g., urology and general surgery, both cranial and spine robotic devices are not emerging and becoming commonly used in neurosurgery. Such devices assist the surgeon in more accurately identifying intracranial lesions, e.g., robotic assisted radiosurgery and placing, for example, pedicle screws. Such applications in the field of neurosurgery have resulted in an explosion of publications regarding this topic over the last several years (McKenzie et al. 2021; Philip et al. 2021).

Herein, the authors have contributed their expertise on the use of robotic technology in neurosurgery. These chapters cover many topics including the use of robotics in endovascular and cerebrovascular surgery, robotics in neuroendoscopy, and surgeon supporting robotics. A chapter devoted to the future of robotics rounds out the offering and reminds us that as technology advances in this realm, greater acceptance and use will most definitely occur. Taken together, this collection of knowledge on this modern topic is timely and will certainly be of interest to neurosurgeons and those interested in robotics in general. As this field is in its infancy, the future is bright for improved accuracy and ease of use as well as additional applications of the technology.

The editors thank each of the contributing authors and hope that this book will spark greater interest in the field of robotics in neurosurgery. We believe that as the surgical microscope exponentially advanced the field of neurosurgery, robotics will, in short order, do the same.

Baghdad, Iraq   Mohammed Maan Al-Salihi
New Orleans, LA, USA   R. Shane Tubbs
Doha, Qatar   Ali Ayyad
Kawasaki, Japan   Tetsuya Goto
Bonn, Germany   Mohammad Maarouf

References

Goodrich JT. History of spine surgery in the ancient and medieval worlds. Neurosurg Focus 2004; 16(1):2.

McKenzie DM, Westrup AM, O'Neal CM, Lee BJ, Shi HH, Dunn IF, Snyder LA, Smith ZA. Robotics in spine surgery: a systematic review. J Clin Neurosci 2021; 89:1–7.

Philipp LR, Matias CM, Thalheimer S, Mehta SH, Sharan A, Wu C. Robot-assisted stereotaxy reduces target error: a meta-analysis and meta-regression of 6056 trajectories. Neurosurgery 2021; 88:222–233.

Acknowledgments

I deeply thank all the book editors, chapter authors, and professors who provided foreword letters. I also thank my friend Dr. Mohaned M. Alazzawi for being supportive and a good advisor. Finally, I can never express enough gratitude to my professor and the dean of my college, Professor Ali K. Alshalchy for being the main source of inspiration for many generations of neurosurgeons.

Mohammed Maan Al-Salihi

I would like to thank my co-editors for their hard work and expertise and the many authors who have contributed to the novelty of this book project. Also, I thank the Department of Neurosurgery at Tulane University School of Medicine and our chair, Dr. Aaron Dumont, for their dedication to academia.

R. Shane Tubbs

I would take this opportunity to thank the authors who have made remarkable contributions to this priceless book. I am also grateful to the co-authors, especially Dr. Mohammed Al-Salihi, for their effort in making this project a success.

Ali Ayyad

Professor Yoshihiro Muragaki, Professor Hiroshi Iseki, and Professor Masakatsu G Fujie who taught me the first steps in robotic neurosurgery research and practice. Dr. Jun Okamoto and Dr. Hideki Okuda with whom we work together on a daily basis.

Tetsuya Goto

I would like to take this opportunity to recognize the help I received in the preparation of the book chapter "Robotics in Stereotactic Neurosurgery" and reviewing the manuscripts of the book.

I am grateful to my loving wife Yaman and my son Abdulrahman who read the manuscript.

Mohammad Maarouf

Contents

Contributors

Narjiss Aji Faculty of Medicine and Pharmacy of Rabat, Mohammed 5 University, Rabat, Morocco

Maryam Sabah Al-Jebur College of Medicine, University of Baghdad, Baghdad, Iraq

Mohammed Maan Al-Salihi College of Medicine, University of Baghdad, Baghdad, Iraq

Darius Ansari Department of Neurosurgery, University of Illinois at Chicago, Chicago, IL, USA

Ali Ayyad Department of Neurosurgery, Saarland University Hospital, Homburg, Germany

Department of Neurosurgery, Hamad General Hospital, Doha, Qatar

Kenza Benkirane Faculty of Medicine and Pharmacy of Fez, University of Sidi Mohamed Ben Abdellah, Fes, Morocco

Joshua D. Burks Department of Neurological Surgery, University of Miami School of Medicine, Miami, FL, USA

Lucas Capo Sagrat Cor University Hospital, Barcelona, Spain

Sorayouth Chumnanvej Neurosurgery Division, Surgery Department, Faculty of Medicine Ramathibodi Hospital, Mahidol University, Bangkok, Thailand

Sandrine de Ribaupierre Department of Clinical Neurological Sciences, Schulich School of Medicine and Dentistry, and Brain and Mind Institute, University of Western Ontario, London, ON, Canada

Francesco Doglietto Neurosurgery, Department of Medical and Surgical Specialties, Radiological Sciences and Public Health, University of Brescia, Brescia, Italy

Fondazione Policlinico Universitario Agostino Gemelli IRCCS, Rome, Italy

Catholic University School of Medicine, Rome, Italy

Roy Eagleson Electrical and Computer Engineering, and Brain and Mind Institute, University of Western Ontario, London, ON, Canada

Fatima Ezzahraa El Idrissi Faculty of Medicine and Pharmacy of Fez, University of Sidi Mohamed Ben Abdellah, Fes, Morocco

Anton Fomenko Section of Neurosurgery, Department of Surgery, Rady Faculty of Health Sciences, University of Manitoba, Winnipeg, MB, Canada

Marco Maria Fontanella Neurosurgery, Department of Medical and Surgical Specialties, Radiological Sciences and Public Health, University of Brescia, Brescia, Italy

Tetsuya Goto Department of Neurosurgery, St. Marianna University School of Medicine, Kawasaki, Kanagawa, Japan

Aria M. Jamshidi Department of Neurological Surgery, University of Miami School of Medicine, Miami, FL, USA

Jesus Lafuente UAB (Autonomous University of Barcelona), Barcelona, Spain

Spine Unit at Hospital del Mar, Barcelona, Spain

Mohammad Maarouf Faculty of Medicine, University of Cologne, Köln, Germany

Department of Neurosurgery, Stereotactic and Functional Neurosurgery, Beta Clinic Bonn, Bonn, Germany

Alba Madoglio Neurosurgery Unit, Department of Neuroscience and Rehabilitation, University of Ferrara, Ferrara, Italy

Ankit I. Mehta Department of Neurosurgery, University of Illinois at Chicago, Chicago, IL, USA

Hajar Moujtahid Faculty of Medicine and Pharmacy of Rabat, Mohammed 5 University, Rabat, Morocco

Clemens Neudorf Movement Disorders and Neuromodulation Unit, Department of Neurology, Charite'—Universitätsmedizin Berlin, Berlin, Germany

Oumaima Outani Faculty of Medicine and Pharmacy of Rabat, Mohammed 5 University, Rabat, Morocco

Elena Roca Neurosurgery, Head and Neck Department, Istituto Ospedaliero Fondazione Poliambulanza, Brescia, Italy

"Technology for Health" Ph.D. Program, University of Brescia, Brescia, Italy

Demitre Serletis Department of Neurosurgery, Cleveland Clinic Foundation, Cleveland, OH, USA

Charles Shor Epilepsy Center, Neurological Institute, Cleveland Clinic, Cleveland, OH, USA

Alejandro M. Spiotta Department of Neurosurgery, Medical University of South Carolina, Charleston, SC, USA

Robert M. Starke Department of Neurological Surgery, University of Miami School of Medicine, Miami, FL, USA

Fabio Tampalini Department of Information Engineering, University of Brescia, Brescia, Italy

R. Shane Tubbs Department of Neurosurgery, Tulane University, New Orleans, LA, USA

Introduction and History of Robotics in Neurosurgery

Anton Fomenko, Fatima Ezzahraa El Idrissi, Narjiss Aji,
Oumaima Outani, Kenza Benkirane, Hajar Moujtahid,
Mohammed Maan Al-Salihi, and Demitre Serletis

1 Introduction

In the current era of the fourth industrial revolution, there is an increasing demand for digitization and automation, with corresponding changes arising in the healthcare landscape. Surgery, which calls for extreme precision and exactness, has particularly benefited from this transition, and robotic surgical techniques are now continually reshaping this field and redefining the ways in which surgeons treat their patients. The first surgical specialty to adopt robotic surgery was neurosurgery; in 1985, a stereotactic biopsy of a deep intracerebral lesion was performed with the guidance of a modified industrial robot, the Programmable Universal Machine for Assembly (PUMA) 200 robotic arm by Unimation [1, 2]. Since this introduction,

A. Fomenko
Section of Neurosurgery, Department of Surgery, Rady Faculty of Health Sciences,
University of Manitoba, Winnipeg, MB, Canada
e-mail: fomenkoa@myumanitoba.ca

F. E. El Idrissi · K. Benkirane
Faculty of Medicine and Pharmacy of Fez, University of Sidi Mohamed Ben Abdellah,
Fes, Morocco
e-mail: kenza.benkirane1@usmba.ac.ma

N. Aji · O. Outani · H. Moujtahid
Faculty of Medicine and Pharmacy of Rabat, Mohammed 5 University, Rabat, Morocco

M. M. Al-Salihi
College of Medicine, University of Baghdad, Baghdad, Iraq

D. Serletis (✉)
Department of Neurosurgery, Cleveland Clinic Foundation, Cleveland, OH, USA

Charles Shor Epilepsy Center, Neurological Institute, Cleveland Clinic, Cleveland, OH, USA

M. M. Al-Salihi et al. (eds.), *Introduction to Robotics in Minimally Invasive
Neurosurgery*, https://doi.org/10.1007/978-3-030-90862-1_1

robotic technology has proved useful and has made its way successfully into the neurosurgical arena.

The field of neurosurgery is well suited to the implementation of robotic surgical techniques. The complex three-dimensional anatomy of the brain includes innumerable interconnected networks with over- and under-lying blood vessel arrays, all of which can be mapped on to a computerized coordinate reference system. The solid density of the skull encasing these delicate cerebral structures, when rigidly fixed in position, serves as a useful stationary reference point for registration and planning [3]. Moreover, the highly technical nature of neurosurgical procedures, including microsurgical approaches and the prolonged duration of cases, means that surgeons are susceptible to fatigue and undesirable tremors during lengthy procedures [4, 5]. It was therefore natural that robotic technology would eventually become established as an adjunct in neurosurgery.

Several different classification schemata are used in medical robotics, based on either the type of interaction between the robot and the surgeon, the technology of the robot itself, or its kinematic specifications. The following are three major categories, stratified by type of interaction with the surgeon [6, 7]:

1. Supervisory Control systems: Widely used in stereotactic and spine surgery, these devices move to a calculated position and reproduce a set of pre-programmed movements. Co-registration with CT and MR brain imaging allows an algorithm planned off-line by the surgeon to be executed autonomously by the robot [2]. The surgeon typically completes the remainder of the procedure without robotic assistance.
2. Dependent or Master–Slave systems: These are used in tele-neurosurgery or settings where the robot is located in challenging environments, and allow the neurosurgeon to maintain full control of the robot's movements in real time [8]. The surgeon receives a live view of the surgical scene via a monitor or eyepieces and manipulates linkage mechanisms online from a control station, which transmits commands to robotic manipulators in the remotely-situated operative suite.
3. Shared-Control systems: These are mixtures of active and passive systems where the surgeon directly interacts with the operative field rather than from a remote console. The clinician's movements are kinematically enhanced or filtered via the shared-control robot to achieve superior precision or haptic control [9].

In this chapter, we present an overview of the history and evolution of robotics in neurosurgery and its current landscape, with a focus on applications in stereotactic surgery and microneurosurgery.

2   The Evolution of Robotics in Stereotactic Surgery

The word "stereotaxy" is a combination of the Greek words *stereos*, meaning three-dimensional, and *taxis*, meaning arrangement [10]. Neurosurgery, as with other surgical disciplines, requires precision of any given intervention and minimization of harm to the patient. In general, stereotactic neurosurgical procedures involve several steps including application of a referential frame-based or frameless system, registration to patient-specific fiducials, and trajectory planning. In addition to the prolonged standing position in the operating theater, the manual setting, numerical input, calibration, and verification of coordinates can all contribute to human error and potential harm to the patient [5, 11]. To tackle those challenges, robotic assistance has been integrated naturally into the neurosurgical realm to improve efficiency of movement, target accuracy, and the overall safety profile of these procedures, among other important advantages [4, 12]. Robotic technologies are now integrated into several fields of neurosurgery including functional neurosurgery, pediatric neurosurgery, radiosurgery, endoscopic skull-base surgery, spine surgery, and epilepsy surgery [7, 13, 14]. A multitude of procedures now rely on such technologies including deep brain tumor biopsies, ventricular cannulation (including endoscopic third ventriculostomy), pedicle screw placement in spinal fixation, laser ablation procedures, deep intraparenchymal/intraventricular hemorrhage evacuation, deep brain stimulation (DBS), and stereoelectroencephalography (SEEG) electrode placement [6, 12].

Historically, localization of a given lesion in the cranium posed a particularly significant challenge. Despite early anthropological and phrenological conceptions, basic mathematical tools were combined with simple machines to generate the first attempts at craniocerebral topography [3]. During the 1860s, Pierre Paul Broca developed a range of special-purpose calipers such as the mandibular goniometer, along with the craniograph and stereograph, to locate essential skull landmarks such as the external occipital protuberance and the glabellum [3]. In 1903, Emil Theodor Kocher, a Swiss physician, developed a refined craniometer that could be applied to heads of various sizes and across any age group to locate intracranial structures such as the Sylvian fissure. This was later used by Harvey Cushing to locate craniocerebral targets [12]. In 1918, the first practical stereotactic frame based on Cartesian coordinates was developed by the mathematician Robert Henry Clarke and the neurosurgeon Sir Victor Alexander Hayden Horsley. It was later adapted for human use by the Canadian neuroanatomist Aubrey Mussen [15]. Although ahead of its time, Mussen's human stereotaxic prototype remained relatively unnoticed. It was not until important modifications to the Horsley-Clarke apparatus were made several decades later, by Henry T. Wycis and Ernest A. Spiegel, that frame-based human stereotactic surgery was formally established in 1947. This ultimately paved the way for the rapid emergence of stereotactic and functional techniques within the field of neurosurgery.

Over the ensuing decades, the emergence of innovative frameless systems and detailed neuroimaging modalities provided neurosurgeons with further possibilities. For example, the implementation of adherent radiolucent fiducials to the skin, or laser registration, has reduced the need for skull-mounted frames and rigid cranial fixation, improving flexibility and patient comfort. In parallel, the development of computed tomography (CT), followed by magnetic resonance imaging (MRI), has been essential for the stereotactic planning of modern-day non-invasive procedures, such as Gamma Knife radiosurgery and high-intensity focused ultrasound, by facilitating the precise targeting of specific brain regions [12].

Specifically focusing on robotic technology, the first robot in stereotactic surgery was the Unimation PUMA 200, used in 1985 to perform a CT-guided brain biopsy, which yielded diagnostic tissue on its first attempt. After proper calibration of the robot, an end-target accuracy of 1.0 mm (with 0.05–0.1 mm repeatability) and a shortened operative time (compared to unassisted frame-based biopsy) were demonstrated [12, 16]. Nevertheless, the lack of medical safety features and inability to compensate for intraoperative brain shift led to the PUMA 200 being discontinued from operative use following its pioneering demonstration [6].

After modern frameless registration with CT imaging was first demonstrated in 1986, robots especially suited for the neurosurgical suite were quickly developed [17]. These revolutionary systems included the Minerva (University of Lausanne, Lausanne, Switzerland); the Zeiss MKM surgical microscope (Carl Zeiss AG, Oberkochen, Germany); the NeuroMaster (Robotic Institute of Beihang University, Beijing, China); and the PathFinder Robot (Prosurgics, Wycombe, UK) [12]. Despite their limited clinical use, these systems spearheaded several important developments such as intraoperative imaging to correct for brain shift, redundant robotic kinematics, and no-go zones to minimize patient injury in the event of a malfunction.

Building on these developments, the neuromate (Renishaw) robot was the first to receive Food and Drug Administration (FDA) approval in 1997 and became the first device to offer both frame-based and frameless stereotactic registration. Early validation studies showed the accuracy of this system to be comparable to conventional manual frame-based and frameless techniques, while reducing operative time in multiple trajectory calculations [12, 18]. Still in active clinical use today, the neuromate has diversified robotic neurosurgery and has completed thousands of SEEG and DBS electrode placements, along with other neurosurgical procedures [12].

In contrast to the conventional robotic arm, the SurgiScope (ISIS SAS) is a ceiling-mounted surgical microscope with robotic capabilities developed in France during the late 1990s [19]. The SurgiScope was the first robotized platform to offer frameless, fiducial-based targeting with pre-operative MRI registration. Many SurgiScope (ISIS SAS) units have been installed worldwide, and the system is popular because of its modular nature and dual use as a microscope with trajectory overlay features.

First introduced by MedTech in 2012, the widely used and now modernized Robotic Stereotactic Assistant (ROSA, Zimmer Biomet) offers two separate platforms: the ROSA ONE Brain and Spine, each of which features built-in stereotactic trajectory assistance. The ROSA Brain has been installed in over 140 hospitals worldwide and utilized in diverse applications including laser ablation of epileptogenic foci, SEEG electrode insertion, shunt placement, cyst aspiration, and endoscopic procedures [12, 20, 21]. The ROSA Spine platform features capabilities such as trajectory assistance with cervical, thoracic, and lumbar transpedicular and vertebral body percutaneous screw placements.

More recently, the miniaturization of motors and electronics systems has allowed more compact, skull-mounted surgical robots to be developed such as the iSYS1

(Medizintechnik GmbH) and the Renaissance (Mazor Robotics) [12]. These robots are establishing themselves as cost-effective and efficient platforms that enable SEEG to be placed safely and accurately, although they require manual repositioning for contralateral-sided procedures. Furthermore, robotic surgical assistance is gaining traction in procedures benefiting from stereotactic trajectories that are customized to individual patient anatomy, such as endoscopic third ventriculostomies and endoscopic pituitary surgery. Platforms such as ROSA enable the surgeon to plan a patient-specific trajectory and simultaneously assist with tremor-free instrument stability and intraoperative trajectory corrections when required [13, 22].

Pediatric neurosurgery has its own distinctive operative challenges owing to the smaller targets and more fragile brains of infants and young children. The experience of using robotic technology in this patient population was well captured by De Benedictis et al. (2017), who assessed 116 children undergoing a series of 128 surgical procedures at the Bambino Gesù Children's Hospital (Rome, Italy) [23]. The authors reported the specific utility of the ROSA device in this young cohort, spanning several types of neurosurgical procedures including stereotactic biopsy, neuroendoscopy, DBS, SEEG electrode placement, and intracystic catheter placement. Only 3.9% of patients had transient postoperative deficits and none sustained any permanent deficit. This high success rate revealed the safety profile of robotic assistance in pediatric neurosurgical patients and demonstrated progressive reduction in operative time with increased system use. Additional prospective studies capturing larger numbers of patients and comparing end-target accuracy and other metrics, including quality of life and implant revision rates, are necessary to confirm these results [23].

A stroke-related procedure within neurosurgery, focusing on intracerebral hemorrhage (ICH) evacuation, has also benefited from robotic stereotactic innovation. Historically, these procedures would conventionally require a craniotomy to access a suitable cortical entry point for removal of a deep-seated hematoma. This invasive procedure has undergone innovations in recent times, facilitated by stereotactic-guided aspiration through a single burrhole. A recent systematic review compared the outcomes of three neuronavigation systems in minimally invasive ICH evacuation: Medtronic AxiEM, Stryker iNtellect, and BrainLab VectorVision [24]. The first of these systems is based on patient registration using electromagnetic stereotaxy, while the latter two are based on optical stereotaxy. Despite their technological differences and the inherent variations in registration, surgical planning, operative setup, and intraoperative use, all three systems were found to yield equivalent results and excellent accuracy for the procedure. The distinct advantages of pinless electromagnetic registration (AxiEM and iNtellect) include its versatility in cases where rigid skull fixation is contraindicated. In this way, the continuous progress of robotics in stereotactic surgery offers enhanced precision and a more conservative, less invasive approach for hemorrhagic stroke management [24].

In summary, over the past three decades, robotics have offered a significant technological contribution to the ever-evolving field of stereotactic neurosurgery, showing promising and safe results and addressing inherent challenges within complex neurosurgical procedures. Most notably, they have revolutionized the concepts of precision and accuracy, reproducibility, indefatigability, and endurance, all challenges faced by the modern-day neurosurgeon.

3   Robotics in Microsurgery

Microneurosurgery has evolved to include the neurosurgical microscope; miniaturized surgical instruments; and the delicate, minimally invasive and non-traumatic maneuvering required to access lesions of the nervous system. Theodore Kurze (1957) was the first neurosurgeon to use the microscope in the operating theater, for removing a neurilemoma of the seventh nerve in a five-year-old patient [25]. Among several subsequent pioneering neurosurgeons at that time, Professor Gazi Yaşargil is widely acknowledged as the most influential neurosurgeon to advance the field of microneurosurgery during the 1960s, developing techniques, microsurgical tools and approaches that have revolutionized the field ever since [26].

Fast-forwarding to the era of modern-day robotic technologies, a number of microsurgical robots have since been introduced into the operating theater. The Robot-Assisted Microsurgery System, or RAMS (NASA, Pasadena, CA), was one of the earliest examples. It comprised a 6-DOF (degrees of freedom) master–slave telemanipulator with programmable controls. In a feasibility study, ten rats underwent carotid arteriotomies in 1 mm diameter arteries that were later closed using either RAMS or the conventional manual technique [27]. The anastomoses were efficiently performed using RAMS, although the surgeons occasionally required external assistance while holding a needle or placing a suture with the robot. The accuracy, technical degree, and ratio error of RAMS and those of conventional techniques were similar. However, RAMS doubled the procedure duration [28, 29].

NeuRobot (Shinshu University School of Medicine, Matsumoto, Japan) was a telecontrolled micromanipulator system made of four main parts: a slave manipulator, a manipulator-supporting device, a master manipulator, and a three-dimensional display monitor [30]. A three-dimensional endoscope and three sets of micromanipulators, each with 3-DOF (rotation, neck swinging, and forward/backward motion), were connected to the slave manipulator. According to one report, NeuRobot was used clinically by neurosurgeons for the partial resection of brain tumors. However, the micromanipulators were limited to a restricted workspace of 10 cubic millimeters, resulting in limited maneuverability and frequent repositioning of the device for larger lesions [28, 29].

The Steady Hand System (Johns Hopkins University, Baltimore, Maryland) is another surgical robotic system developed for enhanced tool manipulation, and is one of the few shared-control surgical robotic systems to have been developed [9]. This device permitted the operator's hand movements to be refined with tremor-filtering functionality, resulting in smoother, dexterity-enhanced motion control of the instrument. Despite the novelty of this machine, the system could not be implemented into more complex interventions (such as anastomoses) owing to a lack of a dimensional scaling function. Despite its apparent benefits, implementation of this system was restricted to retinal microsurgery [6, 28, 29].

The da Vinci telesurgical system (Intuitive Surgical, Sunnyvale, California) is perhaps the most widely-adopted robotics system in medicine, yet its application in neurosurgery has been limited [31]. It comprises a master-slave system involving a stand-alone robotic tower and a master console. A binocular lens and camera system transmits magnified three-dimensional images of the surgical field to the surgeon's control panel, while two or three robotic instrument arms with 6-DOF allow for increased surgical dexterity [32]. A significant advantage of the da Vinci surgical system is the illusion of operating directly on the patient thanks to the anthropomorphic master console with integrated high-resolution twin eyepiece. The da Vinci robot has been used in several surgical fields, notably urology, but some groups have indicated its possible convenience in spinal surgery. To date, it has been used in resection of thoracolumbar neurofibromas, resection of paraspinal schwannomas, and anterior lumbar interbody fusions [33–35]. Because the system incorporates multiple robotic arms instead of a single shaft structure, there is a potential for arm collisions in confined working spaces or volumes. Thus, in narrow neurosurgical operative corridors, these limitations could diminish surgical workflow and therefore pose particular safety issues, limiting the use of the system in microneurosurgical procedures [14, 29].

A revolutionary neurosurgical system that began development in 2001 was the NeuroArm (University of Calgary, Alberta, Canada) [8]. Originally developed to be compatible within an open-bore MRI, it allows for real-time imaging of the surgical field during the procedure. The NeuroArm is a master–slave robot equipped with two robotic arms that can manipulate both conventional and specially-designed microsurgical instruments. The master control station features sensory immersion such as visual, auditory, and haptic feedback to the operator from a remote operative field. The manipulator's arms each have 8-DOF and two force sensors at their extremities. The system also includes end effectors that move in tandem with the operator's hand and can manipulate microsurgical instruments dexterously. It has since been successfully integrated into numerous clinical neurosurgical procedures in a graded fashion, highlighting the important contributions of robotic technology to precision and accuracy in the operating theater [8, 36]. The most recent innovation to the NeuroArm has been neuroArmPLUS[HD], which is a superior neurosurgery-specific haptic device with (7 + 2)-DOF and a serial linkage feature that increases system perceptiveness and is capable of simulating the human hand. A study comparing neuroArmPLUS[HD] to other haptic devices such as Premium (6-DOF, serial linkage design) and Sigma 7 ((6 + 1)-DOF, parallel linkage design) showed that neuroArmPLUS[HD] presented a higher level of performance for angular manipulation, procedure completion duration, force applied, number of clutches and distance covered [29, 37, 38].

In summary, modern-day advances in surgical robotic technology for microsurgery continue to unfold in an interdisciplinary fashion, relying on increased contributions from engineering, physics, and mathematics. Current systems such as the neuroArmPLUS[HD] continue to push the frontiers of what robotic systems can offer to microneurosurgery. In particular, the positive effects on remote surgery, surgical precision, and accuracy, and tremor-free micro-manipulations, are paving the way toward increasingly safer approaches. Nevertheless, newly-emerging robotic systems in microsurgery must continue to address the critical constraints of safety, cost-effectiveness, learning curves in adoption, and space constraints in the operating theater [12, 39], among other limitations in the clinical environment.

4 Conclusions

Innovative technologies have brought a plethora of opportunities to the neurosurgical arena. Specifically, robotic neurosurgery can complement human shortcomings in neurosurgical procedures by diminishing tremors, improving safe surgical access to deep targets, automating serial operative steps, and refining geometric exactness. The contributions of robotic technology to stereotactic neurosurgical and microsurgical procedures continue to unfold and this technology is currently driving a paradigm shift in education and simulation for an entire generation of surgeons. These tools are providing neurosurgeons with greater versatility in exploring and performing more complicated procedures. When combined with future advances in telerobotic surgery and virtual/augmented reality systems, robotic technologies could revolutionize access to care for neurosurgical patients in underdeveloped regions with limited access to resources. There is therefore a clinical need for further refinement of future robotic systems, given the fragility of brain structures and the technical errors potentially inherent in the autonomous functionality of these machines, in a delicate environment where the neurosurgeon has small-to-zero margin of error. More research is required to develop these robotic technologies while concomitantly considering their safety profiles and cost-utilization in the operating theater.

References

1. Marcus HJ, Vakharia VN, Ourselin S, Duncan J, Tisdall M, Aquilina K. Robot-assisted stereotactic brain biopsy: systematic review and bibliometric analysis. Childs Nerv Syst. 2018;34(7):1299–309.
2. Kwoh YS, Hou J, Jonckheere EA, Hayati S. A robot with improved absolute positioning accuracy for CT guided stereotactic brain surgery. IEEE Trans Biomed Eng. 1988;35(2):153–60.
3. Serletis D, Pait TG. Early craniometric tools as a predecessor to neurosurgical stereotaxis. J Neurosurg. 2016;124(6):1867–74.
4. Wang MY, Goto T, Tessitore E, Veeravagu A. Robotics in neurosurgery. Neurosurg Focus. 2017;42(5):3171.
5. Fargen KM, Turner RD, Spiotta AM. Factors that affect physiologic tremor and dexterity during surgery: a primer for neurosurgeons. World Neurosurg. 2016;1(86):384–9.
6. Doulgeris JJ, Gonzalez-Blohm SA, Filis AK, Shea TM, Aghayev K, Vrionis FD. Robotics in neurosurgery: evolution, current challenges, and compromises. Cancer Control. 2015;22(3):352–9.
7. Nathoo N, Cavuşoğlu MC, Vogelbaum MA, Barnett GH. In touch with robotics: neurosurgery for the future. Neurosurgery. 2005;56(3):421–33. discussion 421–33
8. Sutherland GR, Wolfsberger S, Lama S, Zarei-nia K. The evolution of neuroArm. Neurosurgery. 2013;72(Suppl_1):A27–32.

9. Taylor R, Jensen P, Whitcomb L, Barnes A, Kumar R, Stoianovici D, et al. Steady-hand robotic system for microsurgical augmentation. Int J Robot Res. 1999;18(12):1201–10.
10. Grunert P, Keiner D, Oertel J. Remarks upon the term stereotaxy: a linguistic and historical note. Stereotact Funct Neurosurg. 2015;93(1):42–9.
11. Zrinzo L. Pitfalls in precision stereotactic surgery. Surg Neurol Int. 2012;3(Suppl 1):S53–61.
12. Fomenko A, Serletis D. Robotic stereotaxy in cranial neurosurgery: a qualitative systematic review. Neurosurgery. 2018;83(4):642–50.
13. Hoshide R, Calayag M, Meltzer H, Levy ML, Gonda D. Robot-assisted endoscopic third ventriculostomy: institutional experience in 9 patients. J Neurosurg Pediatr. 2017;20(2):125–33. Available from: https://thejns.org/pediatrics/view/journals/j-neurosurg-pediatr/20/2/article-p125.xml
14. D'Souza M, Gendreau J, Feng A, Kim LH, Ho AL, Veeravagu A. Robotic-assisted spine surgery: history, efficacy, cost, and future trends. Robot Surg. 2019;6:9–23.
15. Picard C, Olivier A, Bertrand G. The first human stereotaxic apparatus. The contribution of Aubrey Mussen to the field of stereotaxis. J Neurosurg. 1983 Oct;59(4):673–6.
16. Chen J, Chao L. Positioning error analysis for robot manipulators with all rotary joints. In: 1986 IEEE international conference on robotics and automation proceedings; 1986. p. 1011–6.
17. Roberts DW, Strohbehn JW, Hatch JF, Murray W, Kettenberger H. A frameless stereotaxic integration of computerized tomographic imaging and the operating microscope. J Neurosurg. 1986 Oct;65(4):545–9.
18. Li QH, Zamorano L, Pandya A, Perez R, Gong J, Diaz F. The application accuracy of the NeuroMate robot--a quantitative comparison with frameless and frame-based surgical localization systems. Comput Aided Surg. 2002;7(2):90–8.
19. Deblaise D, Maurine P. Effective geometrical calibration of a delta parallel robot used in neurosurgery. In: 2005 IEEE/RSJ international conference on intelligent robots and systems; 2005. p. 1313–8.
20. Lefranc M, Peltier J. Evaluation of the ROSA™ spine robot for minimally invasive surgical procedures. Expert Rev Med Devices. 2016;13(10):899–906. https://doi.org/10.1080/1743444 0.2016.1236680.
21. Brandmeir NJ, Savaliya S, Rohatgi P, Sather M. The comparative accuracy of the ROSA stereotactic robot across a wide range of clinical applications and registration techniques. J Robot Surg. 2018;12(1):157–63. https://doi.org/10.1007/s11701-017-0712-2.
22. Carrau RL, Prevedello DM, de Lara D, Durmus K, Ozer E. Combined transoral robotic surgery and endoscopic endonasal approach for the resection of extensive malignancies of the skull base. Head Neck. 2013;35(11):E351–8.
23. De Benedictis A, Trezza A, Carai A, Genovese E, Procaccini E, Messina R, et al. Robot-assisted procedures in pediatric neurosurgery. Neurosurg Focus. 2017;42(5):1–12.
24. Chartrain AG, Kellner CP, Fargen KM, Spiotta AM, Chesler DA, Fiorella D, et al. A review and comparison of three neuronavigation systems for minimally invasive intracerebral hemorrhage evacuation. J Neurointerv Surg. 2018;10(1):66–74.
25. Kriss TC, Kriss VM. History of the operating microscope: from magnifying glass to microneurosurgery. Neurosurgery. 1998;42(4):899–907. discussion 907–908
26. Hernesniemi J, Niemelä M, Dashti R, Karatas A, Kivipelto L, Ishii K, et al. Principles of microneurosurgery for safe and fast surgery. Surg Technol Int. 2006;15:305–10.
27. Le Roux PD, Das H, Esquenazi S, Kelly PJ. Robot-assisted microsurgery: a feasibility study in the rat. Neurosurgery. 2001;48(3):584–9.
28. Mitsuishi M, Morita A, Sugita N, Sora S, Mochizuki R, Tanimoto K, et al. Master-slave robotic platform and its feasibility study for micro-neurosurgery. Int J Med Robot. 2013;9(2):180–9.
29. Marcus HJ, Seneci CA, Payne CJ, Nandi D, Darzi A, Yang GZ. Robotics in keyhole transcranial endoscope-assisted microsurgery: a critical review of existing systems and proposed specifications for new robotic platforms. Neurosurgery. 2014;10(1):84–95.
30. Hongo K, Kobayashi S, Kakizawa Y, Koyama J-I, Goto T, Okudera H, et al. NeuRobot: telecontrolled micromanipulator system for minimally invasive microneurosurgery-preliminary results. Neurosurgery. 2002;51(4):985–8. discussion 988

31. Wang MY, Goto T, Tessitore E, Veeravagu A. Introduction. Robotics in neurosurgery. Neurosurg Focus. 2017;42(5):E1.
32. Wedmid A, Llukani E, Lee DI. Future perspectives in robotic surgery. BJU Int. 2011 Sep;108(6 Pt 2):1028–36.
33. Matveeff L, Baste JM, Gilard V, Derrey S. Case report: mini-invasive surgery assisted by Da Vinci® robot for a recurrent paravertebral schwannoma. Neurochirurgie. 2020;66(3):179–82.
34. Moskowitz RM, Young JL, Box GN, Paré LS, Clayman RV. Retroperitoneal transdiaphragmatic robotic-assisted laparoscopic resection of a left thoracolumbar neurofibroma. JSLS. 2009;13(1):64–8.
35. Lee JYK, Bhowmick DA, Eun DD, Welch WC. Minimally invasive, robot-assisted, anterior lumbar interbody fusion: a technical note. J Neurol Surg A Cent Eur Neurosurg. 2013;74(4):258–61.
36. Sutherland GR, Lama S, Gan LS, Wolfsberger S, Zareinia K. Merging machines with microsurgery: clinical experience with neuroArm. J Neurosurg. 2013;118(3):521–9.
37. Morita A, Sora S, Nakatomi H, Harada K, Sugita N, Saito N, et al. Medical engineering and microneurosurgery: application and future. Neurol Med Chir. 2016;56(10):641–52.
38. Baghdadi A, Hoshyarmanesh H, de Lotbiniere-Bassett MP, Choi SK, Lama S, Sutherland GR. Data analytics interrogates robotic surgical performance using a microsurgery-specific haptic device. Expert Rev Med Devices. 2020;17(7):721–30.
39. Fiani B, Quadri SA, Farooqui M, Cathel A, Berman B, Noel J, Siddiqi J. Impact of robot-assisted spine surgery on health care quality and neurosurgical economics: a systemic review. Neurosurg Rev. 2020;43(1):17–25. https://doi.org/10.1007/s10143-018-0971-z.

Robotics in Cerebrovascular and Endovascular Neurosurgery

Aria M. Jamshidi, Alejandro M. Spiotta, Joshua D. Burks, and Robert M. Starke

1 Introduction

Over the past several decades, vascular intervention has experienced a shift toward minimally invasive approaches, which allow for faster and safer treatments than traditional open techniques. Novel endovascular treatment modalities including coiling, embolization, stenting, and more recently thrombectomy have become the standard of care for most vascular pathologies [1]. These techniques have resulted in improved clinical outcomes, with lower rates of morbidity and mortality than classical open vascular reconstruction [2, 3].

As our treatment doctrines have advanced, the role of robotics has concurrently burgeoned in many surgical sub-specialties. Surgical robots have several inherent advantages over human dexterity including fatigue and tremor resistance, greater ranges of axial movement, and the ability to perform fine millimetric movements, which allows for their use in confined body cavities. For example, the da Vinci, one of many commercially available robotic devices, has become ubiquitous in urological surgery because it offers arguably superior outcomes to traditional open methods. The robot facilitates highly precise movements through small incisions, ultimately resulting in improved clinical results, decreased scar tissue, less pain, less bleeding, and an overall shorter recovery period for the patient.

Robotic assistance also benefits the surgeon, relieving the physical demands of surgery by reducing fatigue, enabling it to be executed remotely, and imparting a

A. M. Jamshidi (✉) · J. D. Burks · R. M. Starke
Department of Neurological Surgery, University of Miami School of Medicine, Miami, FL, USA
e-mail: aria.jamshidi@jhsmiami.org; joshua.burks@jhsmiami.org; RStarke@med.miami.edu

A. M. Spiotta
Department of Neurosurgery, Medical University of South Carolina, Charleston, SC, USA
e-mail: spiotta@musc.edu

steadiness that the most trained hand cannot provide. The enhancements that robotic technology has afforded to an array of surgical procedures have had major effects on disease intervention, not least in neurosurgery.

The litany of robotic devices approved by the US FDA for use in neurological surgery includes the ROSA robot (Zimmer Biomet, Warsaw, Indiana) for spine surgery and epilepsy monitoring, the Modus V robotically operate exoscope (Synaptive Medical, Toronto, Canada) for subcortical surgery, and the Renaissance Surgical Guidance Robot (Mazor Robotics, Caesarea, Israel) [4–6].

While interest in the use of robots to improve neurosurgical procedures continues to increase, descriptive reporting and data regarding the role of robotics in cerebrovascular and endovascular neurosurgery remain limited. As clinical technologies in this field are growing rapidly with the development of intrasaccular devices and flow diverting stents for aneurysm treatment, there is a great potential for incorporating robotic technology [7]. In this chapter, we provide a broad review of the current status of robotics in cerebrovascular and endovascular neurosurgery and discuss future directions of this expanding field.

2   Classification of Medical Robots

Two main classification systems, technical and interaction, are commonly used in the literature to describe medical robotic technology. From a technical perspective, medical robots come under one of two headings: passive or active effective modules. In passive effector robotics, the surgeon provides the main action in the intervention; the robot's purpose is to hold fixtures at pre-designated locations to help achieve operative precision and improve the acquisition of a predefined surgical target. In contrast, active effector robotics represents a more nuanced, pivotal, and forward role for the robot in surgical intervention by completing more complex movements. While such robots have greater autonomy, the surgeon still oversees the entirety of the procedure and can intervene when indicated [7, 8].

Medical robots can be further classified by surgeon–machine interaction: supervisory controlled, teleoperate, and shared control systems. Supervisory controlled robots are programmable machines that follow specific movements pre-selected offline by the surgeon. Once the pre-planned movements are arranged, the robot completes these motions autonomously while under surveillance [9]. Teleoperated robots, also known as "master–slave" systems, incorporate a surgical module under direct control by a surgeon. The surgeon gives real time input to a command console, often through a force feedback joystick (master), and the surgical manipulator (slave) executes the actions faithfully. The increasingly popular da Vinci Surgical System (Intuitive Surgical, Sunnyvale, California, USA) is the quintessential example of a teleoperated system [10]. Finally, in a shared control system, the surgeon shares control of the surgical instrument with the robot. The surgeon and robot behave synergistically, the surgeon remaining fully in control while the robot provides "steady hand" manipulation in real time [11].

3 Development of Cerebrovascular and Neuroendovascular Robotic Technology

The development of robotics for use in cerebrovascular and endovascular neurosurgery is still in its infancy. While some technologies have undergone more robust testing than others, several of these modalities are still in experimental stages and do not represent the current standard of care. However, the advanced technologies herein discussed represent promising opportunities for growth and clinical implementation [7].

3.1 Cerebral Angiography

Robotic technology has been expanded and used by several groups to perform diagnostic cerebral angiography. In 2011, Murayama et al. were among the earliest adopters of robotic-assisted angiography, using a multiaxis robotic C arm and a surgical OR table that allowed flexibility in the working position because of its eight-axis design. The system provides three-dimensional angiographic images, creating precise visualization of, and catheter guidance through, tortuous vasculature. The flexible C arm also allows for rapid conversion of endovascular procedures to open surgery without repositioning of the patient. Five hundred and one neurosurgical procedures were successfully conducted with the robotic DSA, including many endovascular cases such as intraoperative angiography and coil embolization [12].

Similarly, Lu et al. described a mechanically propelled master–slave system integrated with a three-dimensional image navigation system controlled remotely by the surgeon [13]. Cerebral angiography was successfully completed in 15 patients without complications. The authors demonstrated that remote-controlled catheter guidance is feasible in cerebrovascular cases and reduces radiation exposure to surgeon and staff alike.

Thereafter, Sajja et al. published their results on ten patients who underwent neuroendovascular procedures using the CorPath GRX robotic assisted platform (Corindus Inc., Waltham, USA), the next-generation system after CorPath 200 (Corindus Inc., Waltham, USA) that was initially designed for interventional cardiology procedures. Seven patients underwent elective diagnostic cerebral angiography, and three underwent carotid artery angioplasty and stenting with the robotic platform. No complications were encountered. However, there was conversion to manual control in three diagnostic cases because of a bovine arch that was not previously known [14]. The CorPath GRX robotic-assisted platform used in this study (Fig. 1) consists of a remote physician unit (Fig. 2) and a bedside unit. The bedside unit comprises an articulated arm, a robotic drive, and a single-use disposable cassette (Fig. 3). The cassette translates real-time commands from the remote physician unit to manipulate the devices. The system allows the guidewire, balloon, or stent catheter to be manipulated with one hand and permits an automatic contrast media injector to be operated with the other [14].

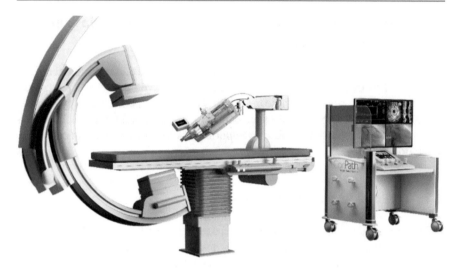

Fig. 1 The CorPathGXR system

The study demonstrated that guidance of the catheter from a remote site is feasible in cerebrovascular cases and could be used in the near future for acute stroke interventions in remote geographical areas.

3.2 Mechanical Carotid Stent Insertion Systems

While robotic assistance for endovascular procedures in the coronary and peripheral vascular arterial system is a rapidly growing field, there remains a dearth of experience and data about its use in the cerebrovascular bed, including the carotid artery. Nogueira et al. described the first case series of four patients who successfully underwent robotically-assisted carotid angioplasty and stenting for treating severe symptomatic carotid stenosis. The authors noted that technical success was achieved in all patients, resulting in resolution of the stenosis with no complications [1].

3.3 Mechanical Coil Insertion Systems

Aside from diagnostic cerebral angiography and carotid stent placement, robotic technology use in neuroendovascular treatment has been limited. However, Pereira et al. recently published the first robotic-assisted therapeutic intervention in a human in which a stent-assisted coiling procedure was used to treat a large basilar aneurysm. All intracranial steps, including stent placement and coil insertion, were performed with assistance from the CorPath Robotic System. At two-week follow-up, a MRI/MR Angiogram (MRA) demonstrated complete obliteration of the

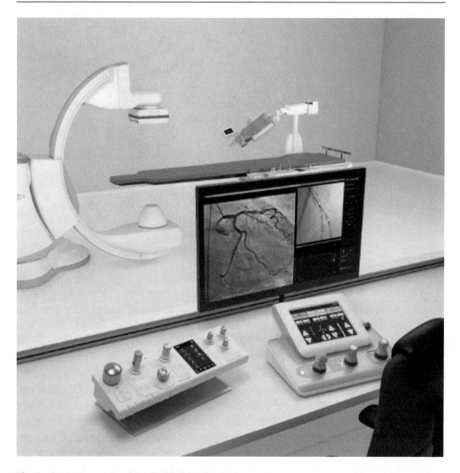

Fig. 2 Control console of the CorPathGRX system

aneurysm. This report represented a major milestone in treating neurovascular disease, opening the doors for remote robotic endovascular treatment [15].

3.4   Robot-Assisted Operating Microscope

Operative microscopes are integral components of the surgical armamentarium for any cerebrovascular interventionalist. Robotic, auto-navigating operating microscopes have recently been developed and evaluated for use in neurosurgical procedures. Bohl et al. examined the use of a robotic, auto-navigating microscope for treating arteriovenous and cavernous malformations. The microscope has several advanced features including the ability to sync with neuronavigation software to align the microscope automatically parallel to a predefined surgical plan, focus on several targets throughout the surgical procedure defined by a particular focal

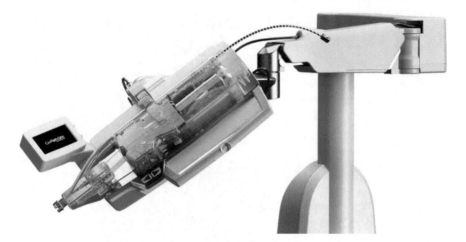

Fig. 3 Robotic arm and cassette of CorPathGRX system

length, and lock on a target defined by the microscope's position. A total of 20 patients were prospectively enrolled, nine of whom harbored vascular lesions. The setup time for the new software interface was less than 1 min in all cases. The authors found the robotic interface to be accurate, reliable, and useful, especially for deep-seated lesions [16].

Similarly, Belykh et al. tested a new robotic visualization platform with novel user-control features, known as the Zeiss Kinevo 900 (Carl Zeiss AG, Oberkochen, Germany), on several anatomical dissections to simulate surgical approaches. They found that the robot improved ocular imaging clarity, improved intraoperative fluorescence visualization, provided better ergonomics, increased the level of intraoperative comfort, and had the potential to affect anatomical instruction positively. While still in its infancy, robotic microscope navigating technology is safe and has the potential to improve surgical efficiency [17].

3.5 Endoscopic Surgical Clipping

Kato et al. published their preliminary findings on the development of a multi-section continuum robot to allow for wide-angled visualization and flexible positioning of the tip of an endoscope during surgical clipping of aneurysms. In this in vitro study, the authors found that the robotic endoscope could potentially allow the surgeon to inspect around and behind aneurysms without displacing other important neurovascular structures, thereby ensuring the safety of the intervention and evaluating the position of the clip to minimize the risk of future rupture [18]. The clinical applications of this technology in vivo could have major effects on the ways in which an array of cerebrovascular pathologies are treated, including arteriovenous malformations and complex aneurysms.

4 Current Technology with Potential Neuroendovascular Applications

Despite advances in robotic-assisted technology for cardiac and peripheral vascular interventions, an FDA-approved robotic platform for neuroendovascular intervention (Table 1) has yet to be approved for mainstream use and dissemination. Britz et al. described a preclinical study investigating off-label use of the CorPath GRX robotic-assisted system in a variety of common neurovascular procedures using an in vitro flow model and a live anesthetized pig. Initially, an access catheter was introduced manually at the equivalent of the common carotid artery in both models. Thereafter, wire and catheters were navigated through the external and internal carotid arteries and the posterior circulation with robotic assistance using 0.014-in. guidewires, 2.4F/1.7F microcatheters, bare-metal stents, and embolic coils. The authors reported successful navigation wiring and deployment of stents and coils in all procedures attempted, with no technical complications. Notably, there was no evidence of extravasation, dissection, or thrombosis on post-procedural angiography [19]. This was the first study to demonstrate that the use of a robotic-assisted platform for neurointervention is safe and feasible.

Subsequently, Desai et al. again used the CorPath GRZ robotic-assisted platform, but this time to embolize intracranial arteriovenous malformations in two anesthetized pigs. After a catheter was introduced manually into the common carotid artery, the robotic system was used to advance it into the ascending pharyngeal artery (APA) toward the rete mirabilis using 0.014 in. guidewires and 2.4F/1.7F microcatheters. A pre-embolization APA run then demonstrated visualization of the

Table 1 Select Food and Drug Administration approved robotic technology in interventional cardiology and radiology with application to endovascular neurosurgery

Robotic system	Manufacturer	Cardiac or peripheral	Intended use	Classification
CorPath GRX robotic system	Corindus	Cardiac and peripheral	Manipulation of guidewires and catheters during percutaneous vascular interventional procedures	Master–slave
Niobe magnetic navigation system	Stereotaxis	Cardiac	Navigation of magnetic devices to direct catheter to desire location in coronary vasculature	Master–slave
Magellan robotic system	Hansen medical	Cardiac and peripheral	Navigation to targets in peripheral vasculature via remotely steerable, multi-directional catheter	Master–slave
Sensei robotic system	Hansen medical	Cardiac	Robotic catheter navigation of coronary vasculature during complex cardiac arrhythmia procedures	Master–slave

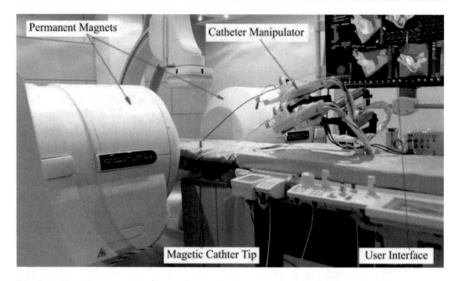

Fig. 4 NiobeVR ES magnetic navigation system. Figure source: Hu X, Chen A, Luo Y, Zhang C, Zhang E. Steerable catheters for minimally invasive surgery: a review and future directions. Comput Assist Surg (Abingdon). 2018;23(1):21–41. (Obtained from "Open Access" sources under a CC-BY license)

rete, a surrogate for an AVM, and thereafter dimethyl sulfoxide was instilled into a microcatheter. A negative roadmap was then created, and Onyx was used to embolize the AVM. The authors reported that all four AVMs were obliterated with no associated vascular injuries or other complications [20].

These and other studies on the Niobe Magnetic Navigating system (Figs. 4 and 5) and Sensei Robotic System (Fig. 6) demonstrate the wide potential applications of robotic platforms in neuroendovascular surgery. The complex and at times tortuous intracranial vascular anatomy has the potential to be navigated carefully by robotically guided millimeter-scale movements in a delicate microcatheter. The ability not only to perform angiography but also to deploy coil stents and embolization material via robotic technology introduces the exciting possibility of also training, proctoring, and performing surgical interventions from long distances [20].

5 Discussion

Robot-assisted cerebrovascular and endovascular neurosurgery.

5.1 Advantages

Robotic-assisted neurointerventions allow for precise device control and deployments, providing additional benefits for patient safety. Minute movements due to physiological tremor are eliminated so navigation is better controlled. The operating team also benefits, avoiding radiation exposure and other occupational hazards.

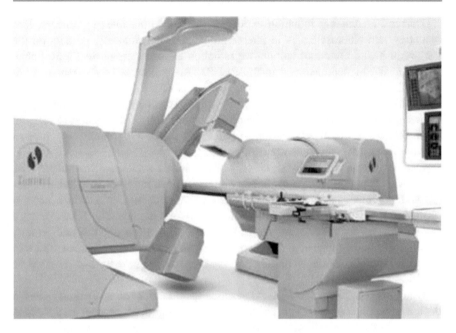

Fig. 5 Niobe by Stereotaxis. Figure source: Beasley RA. Medical robots: Current systems and research directions. J Robot. 2012;2012:1–14. (Obtained from "Open Access" sources under a CC-BY license)

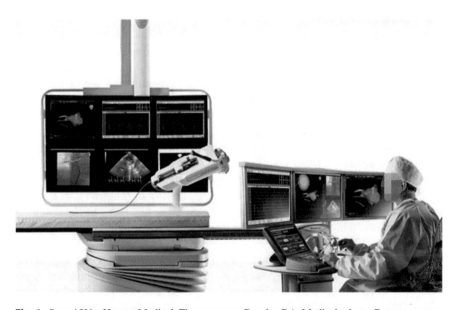

Fig. 6 Sensei X by Hansen Medical. Figure source: Beasley RA. Medical robots: Current systems and research directions. J Robot. 2012;2012:1–14. (Obtained from "Open Access" sources under a CC-BY license)

Decreasing ionizing radiation exposure can reduce the rates of cancers, lens opacities, and atherosclerosis in interventionalists. Unfortunately, no data on the long-term health effects of cumulative radiation exposure are currently available. However, it was demonstrated in the RELID (Retrospective Evaluation study of Lens Injuries and Dose) study that interventionalists have disproportionate rates of cataract-type eye opacities, occurring three times more often than age-matched controlled groups. Robotic assistance can also dramatically reduce musculoskeletal strain related to prolonged wearing of radiation protective garments, which often lead to permanent orthopedic injuries.

One of the most clinically significant innovations associated with endovascular robotics is the potential to perform interventional procedures remotely. Telerobotic-assisted percutaneous coronary intervention was recently successfully accomplished in five patients who were 20 miles away from the operator. If this strategy can be adapted for neurointervention, specifically for mechanical thrombectomy, the clinical ramifications could be revolutionary for acute stroke treatment. Gaps in expertise could be shortened and the speed of reperfusion in remote areas could be significantly improved.

Other benefits of robotic-assisted systems include more controlled and precise device manipulations and deployments. Once reaching the target site, the system is capable of executing extremely stable submillimeter movements. One of the most clinically significant innovations associated with endovascular robotics is the potential to perform interventional procedures remotely.

5.2   Disadvantages

Integration of robots into cerebrovascular and neuroendovascular interventions is not without potential disadvantages and complications. First, cost is a limiting factor with any new technology. The development, manufacturing, and maintenance of advanced robotic systems are expensive, and widespread integration of these technologies would necessitate large investments on the parts of hospitals and healthcare networks [7]. Moreover, training both surgeons and ancillary support staff in the correct usage of new robotic systems can be prolonged and arduous, often involving a steep learning curve. Moreover, the introduction of new technology can alter the workflow in the operating room, specifically as it relates to delaying emergency situations. While remote control of robotic interventional units minimizes the radiation exposure of the surgeon, any delay in transitioning from the endovascular suite to the operating room could have dire consequences for the patient [7].

While robotic neuroendovascular procedures have shown promising initial results, it is of paramount importance to acknowledge that the current robotic systems have been designed for percutaneous cardiovascular and peripheral vascular interventions. Consequently, these platforms are not ideally suited to more complex intracranial techniques, including the ability to manage over-the-wire coaxial systems and other microcatheters safely [21]. Despite the many advances in robotic surgery over the past decade, conversion to manual techniques was required during the critical steps of neuroendovascular procedures such as deployment of a carotid stent and catherization of a bovine arch [14]. These issues question the suitability of this technology in its current state of evolution for conducting these routine procedures.

Finally, an important limitation of robotic assistance is the loss of the tactile feedback critical for performing fine motor tasks. Surgeons rely on this haptic feedback in both vascular and endovascular interventions. Haptic feedback is critical for the safe execution of carotid stenting and coil embolization. Experienced surgeons rely on the ability to sense when they are pushing too hard to deliver a device to a pre-determined landing zone or when a device is not moving in one-to-one synchronicity [22]. Despite the many advances in robotic assistance in neurointerventional procedures, loss of haptics is still a critical limiting factor in dealing with tortuous and delicate intracranial anatomy [21]. However, these limitations are mitigated by the increased control over micromovements that robotic assistance provides using joystick controls and touch screens during stent placement, coil embolization, and diagnostic angiography [22]. This feature is a prime example of the continuing innovation we expect to advance in the future.

The advantages and disadvantages of the robotic technologies mentioned for cerebrovascular and endovascular neurosurgery are shown in Table 2.

6 Future Perspectives

As robotic applications for cerebrovascular and endovascular neurosurgery continue to grow, several factors need to be considered as these technologies are designed, developed, calibrated, and tested. There must be a balance between surgical control and robotic autonomy to allow for safe integration, utilization, and adaptation to constantly evolving surgical conditions. While robotic-assisted devices permit increased accuracy, precision, and seemingly unwavering endurance, they lack the experience, training, and reflective judgment required to make real-time, life-saving surgical decisions, especially in a field as highly technical as vascular neurosurgery [7].

Ultimately, further investigation and improvement of this technology are critical before it can become mainstream. Concerns about robotic-assisted procedures including its complexity, manipulating joysticks instead of catheters, and the additional procedure time can be combated by more formal stimulator training and experience with this technology. The promise of these new innovations for improving the quality and accessibility of cerebrovascular procedures such as thrombectomy for acute stroke is vast [23].

Table 2 Advantages and disadvantages of current robotic technologies for cerebrovascular and endovascular neurosurgery

Author	Type of study	Robotic technology	Pros	Cons
Sajja et al. [14]	Clinical	Master–slave system for catheter guidance	– Precise control and deployment of catheter and stent – Radiation avoidance	– Physician needs to obtain access
Lu et al. [13]	Clinical	Master–slave system for catheter guidance	– Reduction of radiation exposure – Automation of surgical process – Safe	– Inconvenient arrangement of robot and operating table
Murayama et al. [12]	Clinical	Robotic DSA system	– Real-time 3D rotational imaging – Easy conversion of endovascular to "open" procedures – Used in many different neurosurgical procedures – Improved safety	– Intraoperative radiation must be carefully monitored – Lower speed rotation than conventional biplane system – Cost
Kato et al. [18]	Experimental	Multi-section continuum robot	– Larger flexibility in tip positioning than conventional endoscope – Viewing angles up to 180 °	– Only tested in vitro
Bohl et al. [16]	Clinical	Auto-navigating microscope	– Easy integration of software – Quick software setup – Used in many different neurosurgical procedures – Safe	– Tested in small sample size study with single surgeon subjective scoring

[a]*DSA* digital subtraction angiography

7   Conclusions

Robotic technology in cerebrovascular surgery is a burgeoning field still in its infancy. With advances in operative techniques and interdisciplinary collaboration at its peak, there are opportunities and potential for robotics to make meaningful changes in neurointerventional surgery. Technologies under development for cerebrovascular and endovascular neurosurgery include robot-assisted coil placement, angiography, robotic-navigated robotic microscopes, and endoscopic clipping devices, among others. As this discipline continues to advance, it is essential that we proceed in a careful, systematic, and impartial manner that emphasizes patient care, safety, and efficacy.

References

1. Panesar SS, Britz GW. Endovascular robotics: the future of cerebrovascular surgery. World Neurosurg. 2019;129:327–9. https://doi.org/10.1016/j.wneu.2019.06.126.
2. Lanfranco AR, Castellanos AE, Desai JP, Meyers WC. Robotic surgery: a current perspective. Ann Surg. 2004;239(1):14–21. https://doi.org/10.1097/01.sla.0000103020.19595.7d.
3. Tan A, Ashrafian H, Scott AJ, et al. Robotic surgery: disruptive innovation or unfulfilled promise? A systematic review and meta-analysis of the first 30 years. Surg Endosc. 2016;30(10):4330–52. https://doi.org/10.1007/s00464-016-4752-x.
4. Goto T, Miyahara T, Toyoda K, et al. Telesurgery of microscopic micromanipulator system "NeuRobot" in neurosurgery: interhospital preliminary study. J Brain Dis. 2009;1:45–53. https://doi.org/10.4137/jcnsd.s2552.
5. Wolf A, Shoham M, Michael S, Moshe R. Feasibility study of a mini, bone-attached, robotic system for spinal operations: analysis and experiments. Spine (Phila Pa 1976). 2004;29(2):220–8. https://doi.org/10.1097/01.BRS.0000107222.84732.DD.
6. Gonzalez-Martinez J, Bulacio J, Thompson S, et al. Technique, results, and complications related to robot-assisted stereoelectroencephalography. Neurosurgery. 2016;78(2):169–80. https://doi.org/10.1227/NEU.0000000000001034.
7. Menaker SA, Shah SS, Snelling BM, Sur S, Starke RM, Peterson EC. Current applications and future perspectives of robotics in cerebrovascular and endovascular neurosurgery. J Neurointerv Surg. 2018;10(1):78–82. https://doi.org/10.1136/neurintsurg-2017-013284.
8. Nathoo N, Cavusoglu MC, Vogelbaum MA, Barnett GH. In touch with robotics: neurosurgery for the future. Neurosurgery. 2005;56(3):421–33.; discussion 421–33. https://doi.org/10.1227/01.neu.0000153929.68024.cf.
9. Zamorano L, Li Q, Jain S, Kaur G. Robotics in neurosurgery: state of the art and future technological challenges. Int J Med Robot. 2004;1(1):7–22. https://doi.org/10.1002/rcs.2.
10. Avgousti S, Christoforou EG, Panayides AS, et al. Medical telerobotic systems: current status and future trends. Biomed Eng Online. 2016;15(1):96. https://doi.org/10.1186/s12938-016-0217-7.
11. He X, Gehlbach P, Handa J, Taylor R, Iordachita I. Toward robotically assisted membrane peeling with 3-DOF distal force sensing in retinal microsurgery. Annu Int Conf IEEE Eng Med Biol Soc. 2014;2014:6859–63. https://doi.org/10.1109/EMBC.2014.6945204.
12. Murayama Y, Irie K, Saguchi T, et al. Robotic digital subtraction angiography systems within the hybrid operating room. Neurosurgery. 2011;68(5):1427–32.; discussion 1433. https://doi.org/10.1227/NEU.0b013e31820b4f1c.
13. Lu WS, Xu WY, Pan F, Liu D, Tian ZM, Zeng Y. Clinical application of a vascular interventional robot in cerebral angiography. Int J Med Robot. 2016;12(1):132–6. https://doi.org/10.1002/rcs.1650.
14. Sajja KC, Sweid A, Al Saiegh F, et al. Endovascular robotic: feasibility and proof of principle for diagnostic cerebral angiography and carotid artery stenting. J Neurointerv Surg. 2020;12(4):345–9. https://doi.org/10.1136/neurintsurg-2019-015763.
15. Mendes Pereira V, Cancelliere NM, Nicholson P, et al. First-in-human, robotic-assisted neuroendovascular intervention. J Neurointerv Surg. 2020;12(4):338–40. https://doi.org/10.1136/neurintsurg-2019-015671.rep.
16. Bohl MA, Oppenlander ME, Spetzler R. A prospective cohort evaluation of a robotic, auto-navigating operating microscope. Cureus. 2016;8(6):e662. https://doi.org/10.7759/cureus.662.

17. Belykh EG, Zhao X, Cavallo C, et al. Laboratory evaluation of a robotic operative microscope - visualization platform for neurosurgery. Cureus. 2018;10(7):e3072. https://doi.org/10.7759/cureus.3072.
18. Kato T, Okumura I, Song SE, Hata N. Multi-section continuum robot for endoscopic surgical clipping of intracranial aneurysms. Med Image Comput Comput Assist Interv. 2013;16(Pt 1):364–71. https://doi.org/10.1007/978-3-642-40811-3_46.
19. Britz GW, Tomas J, Lumsden A. Feasibility of robotic-assisted neurovascular interventions: initial experience in flow model and porcine model. Neurosurgery. 2020;86(2):309–14. https://doi.org/10.1093/neuros/nyz064.
20. Desai VR, Lee JJ, Tomas J, Lumsden A, Britz GW. Initial experience in a pig model of robotic-assisted intracranial arteriovenous malformation (AVM) embolization. Oper Neurosurg (Hagerstown). 2020;19(2):205–9. https://doi.org/10.1093/ons/opz373.
21. Nogueira RG, Sachdeva R, Al-Bayati AR, Mohammaden MH, Frankel MR, Haussen DC. Robotic assisted carotid artery stenting for the treatment of symptomatic carotid disease: technical feasibility and preliminary results. J Neurointerv Surg. 2020;12(4):341–4. https://doi.org/10.1136/neurintsurg-2019-015754.
22. Albuquerque FC, Hirsch JA, Chen M, Fiorella D. Robotics in neurointervention: the promise and the reality. J Neurointerv Surg. 2020;12(4):333–4. https://doi.org/10.1136/neurintsurg-2020-015955.
23. Rabinovich EP, Capek S, Kumar JS, Park MS. Tele-robotics and artificial-intelligence in stroke care. J Clin Neurosci. 2020;79:129–32. https://doi.org/10.1016/j.jocn.2020.04.125.

Robotics in Stereotactic Neurosurgery

Mohammad Maarouf and Clemens Neudorf

1 Introduction

The problem of accessing intracranial targets accurately and reliably for surgical intervention has occupied neurosurgeons ever since the establishment of stereotactic neurosurgery early in the twentieth century. Initial targeting approaches proposed by Horsley and Clarke in 1908 relied on bony landmarks to locate deep brain structures that had proved suitable for surgical interventions in animals [1]. However, their application to humans, involved great variability, ultimately entailing insufficient accuracy for human stereotactic surgery. Building on these initial targeting strategies and driven by the introduction of X-ray imaging for surgical planning, Spiegel and Wycis devised their own stereotactic apparatus in 1947, heralding the era of imaging-guided stereotaxy [1]. By visualizing the third ventricle directly using pneumoencephalography and later ventriculography, they could target the basal ganglia and their associated pathways indirectly, allowing them—for the first time—to intervene deep within the human brain safely and accurately. Their technological success was also reflected in what at the time was a comparatively low operative mortality rate of 2%. This encouraged wide adoption of the Spiegel–Wycis system, sparking further advances in stereotactic techniques in neurosurgery [2]. Returning from a visit to Spiegel and Wycis at Temple Medical School in

M. Maarouf (✉)
Faculty of Medicine, University of Cologne, Köln, Germany

Department of Neurosurgery, Stereotactic and Functional Neurosurgery, Beta Clinic Bonn, Bonn, Germany

C. Neudorf
Movement Disorders and Neuromodulation Unit, Department of Neurology, Charite'—Universitätsmedizin Berlin, Berlin, Germany

© The Author(s), under exclusive license to Springer Nature Switzerland AG 2022
M. M. Al-Salihi et al. (eds.), *Introduction to Robotics in Minimally Invasive Neurosurgery*, https://doi.org/10.1007/978-3-030-90862-1_3

Philadelphia, Lars Leksell designed the first arc-centered apparatus in 1948. Given that the spatial coordinates of the frame indicated the center of a semicircular arc, insertion of surgical probes along any angle allowed deep brain structures to be targeted reliably. Many other groups introduced alternative systems in subsequent years including Talairach in Paris [3], Riechert and Mundinger in Germany [4], and Bailey and Stein in the USA [5].

Supported by technological advances in neuroimaging, which saw the introduction of computed tomography (CT) and magnetic resonance imaging (MRI), and—equally important—the development of fiducial systems that served as reliable reference measures for translating targeting coordinates into the human brain, imaging-guided stereotactic surgery provided novel, minimally invasive opportunities for diagnosing and managing intracranial pathologies [6, 7]. In recent years, stereotaxy has advanced rapidly, extending into the fields of movement disorders, epilepsy, psychiatric diseases, pain and neoplastic diseases of the nervous system. However, with a growing indication spectrum, the complexity of surgical interventions and the surgeon's requirements for precise and reliable tools increases as well. This holds especially true for complex clinical procedures such as stereoencephalography (SEEG), which entails the implantation of up to 10–20 recording electrodes in one patient [8]. Here, the calculation and conversion of coordinates to the stereotactic frame can prove cumbersome and are liable to both human and mechanical error. In addition, the duration of surgical procedures drastically increases with complexity, exposing patients to surgical risks and complications.

In recent years, robotic stereotaxy has emerged as a fast, accurate, and reliable alternative to established stereotactic guiding devices. Following their first introduction in 1985, robotic systems have now reached a level of sophistication that can be considered equal if not superior to conventional approaches [9–12]. As a result, the use of robotic systems has expanded dramatically in operating rooms around the world and has become a mainstay in complex stereotactic procedures such as tumor biopsies, deep brain stimulation, radiosurgery, SEEG, ventricular catheter placement, and laser ablative procedures. While a wide range of surgical robots has been prototyped throughout the years, only a selected few have gained FDA/CE approval and are applied in vivo today.

1.1 Early Robotic Stereotactic Systems

The first application of robotic devices in stereotaxy can be traced back to Kwoh et al., who in 1985 employed an industrial robot, the PUMA 200 (Staubli International AG, Pfaffikon, Switzerland), to perform a brain biopsy [13]. Originally used in the automotive industry, the PUMA 200 featured a single robotic arm with six degrees of freedom, including an articulator and an effector. The robot was connected to a CT scanner, wherein the patient's head was secured in a stereotactic frame. Following imaging and trajectory planning, the robot was engaged and used to align a biopsy cannula automatically along the predefined surgical trajectory. The cannula was then guided by the neurosurgeon to retrieve the diagnostic tissue.

However, owing to technical limitations and mounting safety concerns in the wake of the first procedure, implementation of the PUMA 200 for surgical purposes was eventually discontinued. Nevertheless, the demonstration that robot-assisted stereotaxy was feasible and had enjoyed early success served as grounds for developing robotic systems specifically dedicated to neurosurgery [14].

Following several years of unsuccessful implementation, the NeuroMate (Integrated Surgical Systems, ISS now Renishaw) was the first neurosurgical robot to receive FDA approval in 1997 and the first commercially available robotic system. Providing the possibility of frame-based and frameless registration, case series of robot-assisted brainstem biopsies reported successful histological diagnosis at the first attempt with an 86% success rate. However, the authors also reported transient and permanent neurological deficits in 13% and 6% of patients, respectively [15]. The robot was also deployed for taking pineal biopsies, yielding a diagnostic rate of 99% with transient side effects as low as 6% [16]. The NeuroMate reached another landmark in 2005 with the first reported robot-guided SEEG electrode implantation in the presurgical evaluation of epilepsy. In this retrospective study a total of 42 electrodes were successfully implanted in 17 out of 211 patients [17].

1.2 Current Robotic Stereotactic Systems

Current robotic systems enable automated stereotaxy to be performed with high accuracy and reliability and are rapidly becoming a mainstay in complex stereotactic procedures such as deep brain stimulation (DBS), stereoelectroencephalography (SEEG), and stereotactic laser ablation/MRI-guided interstitial laser thermotherapy (MRgLITT) [9, 11, 12, 18–20].

Several FDA/CE approved robotic stereotaxy devices are currently available, including the NeuroMate robotic system (Renishaw), the ROSA ONE Brain robotic platform (Zimmer Biomet/MedTech, USA/Montpellier, France), and the Stealth Autoguide cranial robotic guidance platform (Medtronic).

The principal applications of stereotactic neurosurgery using robots are discussed below.

2 Robot-Assisted Stereotactic Deep Brain Stimulation

Deep brain stimulation (DBS) constitutes an effective treatment for a broad range of movement disorders and psychiatric diseases. During surgery, leads are advanced deep into eloquent brain structures to apply electric currents to the surrounding brain tissue [21]. Given that clinical outcome correlates strongly with proper lead placement, high precision and accuracy are imperative during electrode implantation [22, 23]. Specifically, it was shown that lead displacement with lateral deviations ≥ 1.40 mm may be associated with unfavorable spread of electrical current to adjacent eloquent areas leading to reduced therapeutic benefit and stimulation-induced side effects that could potentially rule chronic stimulation impossible [24].

While directional leads have been shown to account for slight electrode misplace-ments and increase the therapeutic window of stimulation, Steigerwald et al. [24] emphasized that use of this novel technology "must never be an excuse for lowering the surgical standard and precision of surgical lead placement." Thus, accurate lead placement constitutes the strongest predictor for treatment success in the field of DBS.

Inaccurate electrode implantation may not only be associated with suboptimal stimulation effects, but has the potential to significantly extend the duration of sur-gical procedures. This has severe ramifications on the patient comfort and safety during surgery, increasing the risk of intraoperative complications [25]. Given that patients are typically awake during surgery prolonged surgical procedures may impose a great degree of stress on the patient, which in turn may yield insufficient results during intraoperative stimulation testing.

Given their effective integration into the surgical workflow and improved accu-racy robot-guided DBS has the potential to improve surgical outcome while reduc-ing the duration of surgery. In the following sections we describe our experience with the ROSA Brain (Zimmer Biomet/MedTech, USA/Montpellier, France), one of the most frequently employed stereotactic robots, which has been employed in combination with the O'arm (Medtronic, Minneapolis, MN, USA) since 2015. ROSA Brain features a robotic arm with six degrees of freedom and incorporates a haptic system that allows manual adjustments of the robotic arm. Moreover, the robot is able to perform independent movements under physician supervision.

2.1   Stereotactic Planning and Surgical Procedure

During the preoperative course, three-dimensional, magnetic resonance imaging (MRI) scans were performed in coronal and axial sections using a 1.5 T clinical MRI system (Philips Gyroscan Intera, Philips Ltd., Best, the Netherlands). On the day of surgery, a Leksell series G stereotactic frame (Elekta, Stockholm, Sweden) was attached to the patient's head. A stereotactic, contrast-enhanced computed tomography (CT) scan (SOMATOM Definition Flash, Siemens, Erlangen, Germany) was then obtained in axial sections [9]. Imaging parameters for the CT scan were: matrix size 512×512, field of view 300 mm, slice distance 1 mm, volt-age 100 kV, current-time product 350 mAs and kernel H31s. Stereotactic transfor-mation, image fusion with MRI scans and DBS planning were then realized using the robot planning software Rosanna v2.5.8. (Medtech, Montpellier, France). After target verification the surgical plan was digitally transferred to the robot, and frame-based registration was performed using the robot's haptic capabilities [26]. Registration was only deemed successful if accuracy was below 0.40 mm. In cases where this value was exceeded the robotic system was reset and registration was repeated. Following registration, entry points were identified bilaterally either using the non-sterile pointer or the robot's laser probe. The scalp was subse-quently shaved and following sterile draping two craniostomies were performed at each previously marked entry point, respectively. For electrode implantation, the robotic arm was equipped with a Ben's gun and aligned with the previously planned trajectory. Importantly, the robotic arm was placed at a predefined distance from the target taking into account electrode length. The lead was implanted manually by the neurosurgeon after the lead path was paved with a rigid cannula. Once the electrode was placed within the predefined target, accurate lead placement was confirmed intraoperatively using flat panel CT (fpCT) scans employing the O'arm (Medtronic Inc., Minneapolis, MN, USA) (Fig. 1). After successful intraoperative clinical testing the lead was anchored at the skull and the process was repeated on the contralateral side.

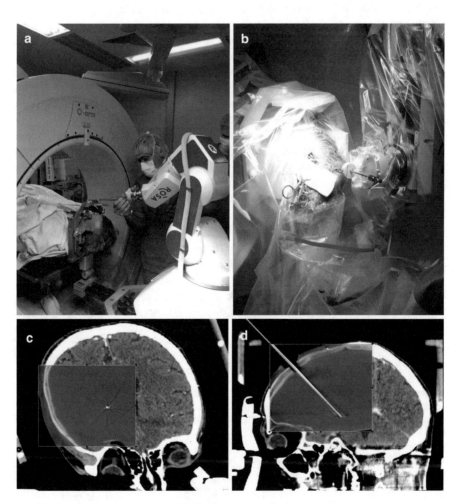

Fig. 1 ROSA (Zimmer Biomet/MedTech, USA/Montpellier, France) frame-based registration using the robot's haptic capabilities (**a**). Image (**b**) demonstrates robot-assisted stereotactic biopsy. Accurate lead placement verified intraop. on O'arm (Medtronic) flat-panel-detector based CT (fpCT) scans: (**c**) perpendicular, (**d**) parallel

2.2 Accuracy and Time-Efficiency of Robot-Assisted Stereotactic DBS

To investigate the efficacy of robot-assisted DBS we compared the ROSA Brain (Zimmer Biomet/MedTech, USA/Montpellier, France) to a conventional stereotactic guiding system, the modified Riechert–Mundinger (RM) stereotactic apparatus (Inomed, Emmendingen, Germany). In total, we evaluated 40 patients who underwent robot-guided electrode implantation for therapy-refractory movement disorders and psychiatric diseases to 40 conventionally implanted patients. To ensure comparability across cohorts and reduce potential biases induced by patient demographics we matched each cohort based on age, gender, underlying disease, DBS target, and number of implanted leads.

Surgery could be performed successfully in all patients (n = 160 leads) without intraoperative complications such as intracranial hemorrhage and lead dislocation. Postoperative comparison of electrode deviations from the originally planned trajectory revealed a mean radial error of 1.11 ± 0.56 mm (range: 0.10–2.90 mm) for the RM-guided DBS, and 0.76 ± 0.37 mm (range: 0.17–1.52 mm) for robot-guided DBS (Fig. 2). Differences between both groups were highly significant ($p < 0.001$) revealing an overall greater variance in the RM-cohort as compared to robot-guided DBS. Taken together, our results suggest that robot-assisted surgery is (1) more accurate than conventional DBS and (2) features greater consistency across procedures. These findings are in accordance with previously reported studies investigating the accuracy of frame-based robot-guided lead implantation. Using the ROSA Brain (Zimmer Biomet/MedTech, USA/Montpellier, France) with a Leksell G frame, Lefranc et al. reported a mean radial error of 0.81 ± 0.39 mm [26]. Similarly, Li et al. reported target error values of 0.86 ± 0.32 mm using the NeuroMate (Renishaw) in combination with a Fischer Frame (Fischer Surgical Inc., Imperial, Missouri) [27].

Comparison of operation times across surgical implantation modalities revealed a statistically significant difference, indicating a mean reduction of implantation time by at least 1 h during robot-guided DBS [9]. Furthermore, image quality was

Fig. 2 Accuracy of robot-guided vs. conventional lead implantation. The box plot features the radial errors (lateral deviation) between final and planned trajectories. Implantation accuracy differed significantly between the two modalities ($p < 0.05$). Note the increased variance of Riechert–Mundinger (RM) guide DBS. Adopted with permission from Neudorfer et al. (2018) [9]

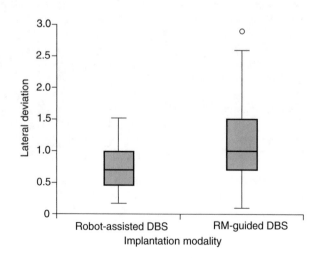

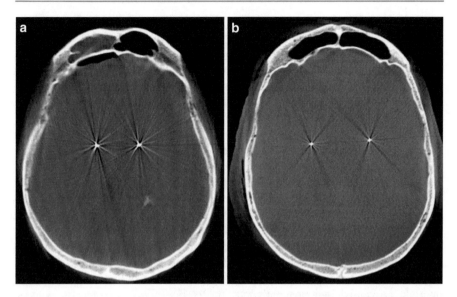

Fig. 3 Comparison of imaging quality across implantation modalities during intraoperative electrode verification. (**a**) Conventional DBS is associated with distinct metal artifacts caused by both the frame and aiming bow of the Riechert–Mundinger (RM) system. (**b**) Since robot-guided DBS does not rely on mechanical guiding devices, metal artifacts can be reduced effectively. Only two carbon rods that rigidly connect the stereotactic frame to the robotic system are located within the beam path. However, this has negligible effects on image quality. Adopted with permission from Neudorfer et al. (2018) [9]

drastically improved during robot-assisted DBS. This is owing to the fact that no guiding device was located along the beam path during fpCT. In conventional DBS this is unavoidable, yielding an increased amount of artifacts during lead placement verification (Fig. 3). Importantly, the reduction of metal artifacts during robot-guided DBS offers the potential to minimize the effective radiation doses applied to the patient's head during surgery [9].

Taken together, the findings of our study suggest that robot-assisted DBS surgery can be considered superior to conventional lead implantation in terms of accuracy and reliability. Clinically meaningful deviations were never attained during robot-guided DBS. Hence, robot-assisted DBS can be considered an appropriate alternative to mechanical guiding devices.

3   Robot-Assisted Stereotactic Diagnosis and Therapy for Epilepsy

3.1   Conventional Surgery for Epilepsy

Epilepsy surgery constitutes an effective therapeutic option for treating refractory epilepsy. Wiebe et al. reported 64% seizure freedom in a randomized trial (RCT) of surgery for temporal lobe epilepsy (TLE) [28]. Thus, surgery was recommended as the treatment of choice for drug-resistant TLE [29]. A second RCT of surgery for TLE, the Early Randomized Surgical Epilepsy Trial (ERSET), designed to operate within 2 years of failure of two appropriate drug trials, reported 85% seizure freedom. In addition, health-related quality of life and measures of socialization were better in the surgical than the medical arm [30]. A recent RCT of pediatric epilepsy surgery from India highlighted the importance of epilepsy surgery in children [31].

3.2   Definition of the Epileptogenic Zone

For presurgical definition of the epileptogenic zone (EZ), non-invasive investigations are sufficient in most cases [32, 33]. However, in 25–50% of subjects, identification of the EZ cannot be achieved by non-invasive means, necessitating the use of intracranial stereoelectroencephalography (SEEG) [17, 34, 35].

Robotic systems have been effectively implemented as a minimally invasive and highly accurate means for the diagnosis and therapy of epilepsy. Indeed, the automated workflow and the ease of implementation with respect to the employment of multiple sequential and noncontiguous trajectories allow significantly reduced operative times while effectively maintaining accuracy and precision [36].

Accuracy data of SEEG electrode placements have been published for Neuromate, ROSA, and iSYS1. A meta-analysis of accuracies of implantation methods revealed significant heterogeneity among studies, mainly because different accuracy measures were used [11]. Robotic guidance achieved a median 0.78 mm entry point and 1.77 mm target point error, compared to a median 1.43 mm entry point and 2.69 mm target point error with manual Talairach frame placement [37]. The complication rate from SEEG is low. The overall morbidity rate has been reported as 1.3% per patient, equating to a risk of 1 in 287 electrodes. Hemorrhage occurred in 1% of patients [38].

3.3   Robot-Guided MRgLITT

MRI-guided laser interstitial thermal therapy (MRgLITT) has pivotal advantages owing to the combination of narrow-caliber cooled-fibers for laser interstitial thermal therapy and magnetic resonance thermography for non-invasive real-time imaging of tissue temperature. Furthermore, robotic stereotaxy and laser technology can be combined to provide a minimally invasive therapy, giving surgeons a method for ablating tissue across a number of subspecialties, including epilepsy and neurooncology, with a potentially faster workflow, higher accuracy, and reliability than frame-based or frameless systems.

Two commercial platforms using this technology are currently available for central nervous system applications, NeuroBlate (Monteris) and Visualase (Medtronic). In MRgLITT the goals are complete ablation of the epileptogenic zone while avoiding injury to uninvolved and eloquent structures. (Fig. 4) demonstrates a representative case of mesial temporal lobe epilepsy treated with robot-guided MRgLITT. Wu et al. published the first multicenter study of LITT for MTLE and the largest LITT series of 234 patients in 2019 with long-term follow-up of seizure outcome. At

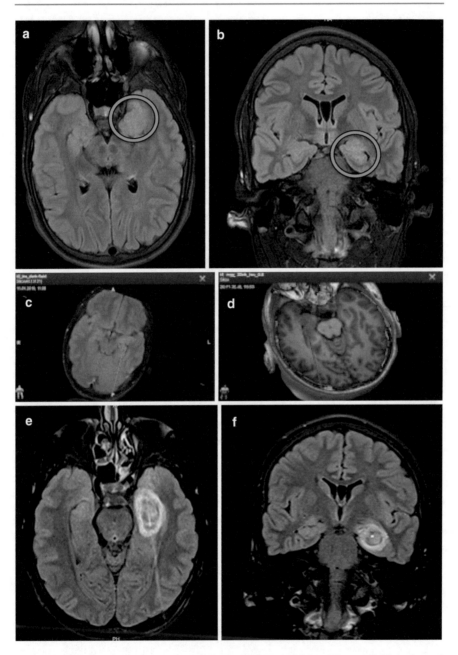

Fig. 4 LITT for Mesial Temporal Lobe Epilepsy (MTLE). Axial (**a**) and coronal (**b**) sections of T2-weighted MRI scans obtained in the preoperative course reveal a left-sided hippocampal sclerosis in a patient suffering from therapy-refractory TLE. Trajectory planning (**c, d**). Postoperative T2w scans featuring the LITT ablation zone in axial (**e**) and coronal (**f**) sections

latest follow-up of at least 1 year (mean: 30 ± 14 months, 12–75 months), 58.0% of the cohort achieved Engel I outcomes, and 76.9% achieved either Engel I or II outcomes. The persistence of this seizure outcome at 2 years underlines the durability of the therapy [18]. In a nonrandomized comparison, MRgLiTT for MTLE has demonstrated similar outcomes as open surgical techniques with respect to efficacy of seizure control while minimizing collateral injury [18, 39].

In addition, robot guided MRgLITT provides a number of benefits, including those associated with minimally invasive techniques such as smaller incisions and reduced hospitalization time. Complication rates of open temporal lobectomy and the incidence of visual field deficits [40, 41] are reduced after application of robot-guided MRgLITT, and neuropsychological deficits in naming and object recognition are lower and patient experience is improved [39]. Thus, MRgLITT has the potential to gain wider acceptance than the open surgical techniques.

4   Robot-Assisted Stereotactic Brain Biopsy

Brain biopsy was the first stereotactic procedure adopted for surgical robotics, performed in 1985 by Kwoh et al. on a 52-year-old man who was diagnosed with a suspicious intra-cerebral lesion [14]. As it is important to ensure that tissue samples are obtained from the biologically most active and prognostically relevant parts of the tumor, incorporation of structural (MRI) and metabolic (PET) imaging data in the planning of a stereotactic biopsy can be essential, and they minimize the risk of under-grading, misdiagnosis, and under-treatment of heterogeneously composed gliomas [42, 43]. Thus, the use of multiple trajectories can be beneficial and is indicated. Reflecting the need for precise and comprehensive retrieval of representative tissue for detailed histological and molecular genetic examination, stereotactic biopsies constitute the most prevalent indication for robotic systems today, over 500 patients having undergone this procedure to date. In accordance with this notion, all commercially available stereotactic robots have been used for this procedure, NeuroMate (Renishaw) and ROSA (ZimmerBiomet) leading the total number of studies reporting their successful deployment.

Lefranc et al. evaluated the ROSA® robot and found that the accuracy of frame-based registration (0.81 mm) and bone-fiducial registration (0.7 mm) was greater in comparison to surface registration (1.22 mm). Furthermore, the authors found that MRI as the reference image was significantly less accurate overall, probably because of distortion in the MRI system [26].

4.1   Diagnostic Yield and Complications

To date, only retrospective cases series have been published and reported on the diagnostic accuracy of robot-assisted stereotactic brain biopsy. One of the largest studies was that of Lefranc et al. who reported on a consecutive series of 100 cases that under-went frameless robotic stereotactic biopsies using the ROSA system. Histological diagnoses were established in 97% of patients. No mortality or permanent morbidity related to surgery was observed. Six patients experienced transient neurological worsening. Six cases of bleeding within the lesion or along the biopsy trajectory were detected on postoperative CT scans, but were associated with transient clinical symptoms in only two cases [20]. Similar results were reported by Zanello et al. who found a high diagnostic yield of 98.7% in a total of 377 cases [44].

Marcus et al. undertook a systematic review and bibliometric analysis of the literature on robot-assisted stereotactic brain biopsy in 2018. Six studies reported on the ROSA® robot, two reported on the NeuroMate® robot, while the remaining studies investigated other robotic systems. The diagnostic biopsy rate ranged from 75% to 100% in individual series. In contrast, the pooled analysis achieved a diagnostic accuracy of 95% of procedures. Fewer than 1% of patients had a significant postoperative hematoma or permanent neurological deficit [45].

5 Perspective

The combination of accurate, reliable, and automated stereotaxy with image and haptic guidance holds the potential to expand the spectrum of minimally invasive procedures. First reports about new indications have already been published. These include LITT for treating brain tumors and metastases [46], robotic-assisted stereotactic internal shunting of surgically inaccessible brain cysts [47], robot-guided ventriculo-peritoneal shunting in slit-like ventricles [48], clinical application of neurosurgical robot in intracranial Ommaya reservoir implantation [49], experimental procedures such as implantation of convection enhanced drug delivery catheters [50], and robotic-assisted stereotactic iodine 125 seeds implantation for interstitial irradiation of brain tumors and metastases (submitted).

6 Conclusion

Numerous studies demonstrate high accuracy and reliability in robotic-assisted stereotactic neurosurgery, along with shorter operative times, excellent surgical performance, and desirable clinical outcomes. Thus, robotic systems are rapidly becoming a mainstay in complex stereotactic procedures such as brain biopsy, deep brain stimulation (DBS), stereo-electro-encephalography (SEEG), and stereotactic laser ablation/MRI-guided interstitial laser thermotherapy (MRgLITT). New applications are already started and undergoing clinical evaluation. Further studies with large numbers of patients are required.

References

1. Spiegel EA, Wycis HT, Marks M, Lee AJ. Stereotaxic apparatus for operations on the human brain. Science (80-). 1947;106(2754):349–50. https://www.sciencemag.org/lookup/doi/10.1126/science.106.2754.349
2. Lozano AM, Gildenberg PL, Tasker RR. In: Lozano AM, Andres M, Gildenberg PL, Tasker RR, editors. Textbook of stereotactic and functional neurosurgery. 2nd ed. Berlin, Heidelberg: Springer; 2009.

3. Mazoyer B. Jean Talairach (1911–2007): a life in stereotaxy. Hum Brain Mapp. 2008;29(2):250–2. http://doi.wiley.com/10.1002/hbm.20473
4. Riechert T, Mundinger F. Beschreibung und Anwendung eines Zielgerätes für stereotaktische Hirnoperationen (II. Modell). In: Röntgendiagnostische Probl bei intrakraniellen Geschwülsten. Berlin, Heidelberg: Springer; 1955. p. 308–37. http://link.springer.com/10.1007/978-3-662-25077-8_45. Accessed 13 Oct 2016.
5. Rahman M, Murad GJA, Mocco J. Early history of the stereotactic apparatus in neurosurgery. Neurosurg Focus. 2009;27(3):1. https://thejns.org/view/journals/neurosurg-focus/27/3/article-pE12.xml
6. Schulder M, Jarchin L. MRI in image guided surgery. In: Lozano AM, Gildenberg PL, Tasker RR, editors. Textbook of stereotactic and functional neurosurgery. 2nd ed. Berlin, Heidelberg: Springer; 2009. p. 599–617. http://link.springer.com/10.1007/978-3-540-69960-6_39.
7. Perry JH, Rosenbaum AE, Lunsford DL, Swink CA, Zorub DS. Computed tomography-guided stereotactic surgery. Neurosurgery. 1980;7(4):376–81. https://academic.oup.com/neurosurgery/article-lookup/doi/10.1227/00006123-198010000-00011
8. Cardinale F, Rizzi M, Vignati E, et al. Stereoelectroencephalography: retrospective analysis of 742 procedures in a single Centre. Brain. 2019;142(9):2688–704. https://academic.oup.com/brain/article/142/9/2688/5532295
9. Neudorfer C, Hunsche S, Hellmich M, El Majdoub F, Maarouf M. Comparative study of robot-assisted versus conventional frame-based deep brain stimulation stereotactic neurosurgery. Stereotact Funct Neurosurg. 2018;96:327–34. https://doi.org/10.1159/000494736.
10. Bradac O, Steklacova A, Nebrenska K, Vrana J, De Lacy P, Benes V. Accuracy of varioguide frameless stereotactic system against frame-based stereotaxy: prospective, randomized, single-center study. World Neurosurg. 2017;104:831–40. https://doi.org/10.1016/j.wneu.2017.04.104.
11. Vakharia VN, Sparks R, O'Keeffe AG, Rodionov R, Miserocchi A, Mcevoy A, et al. Accuracy of intracranial electrode placement for stereoencephalography: a systematic review and meta-analysis. Epilepsia. 2017;58:921–32. https://doi.org/10.1111/epi.13713.
12. Mirzadeh Z, Chen T, Chapple KM, Lambert M, Karis JP, Dhall R, et al. Procedural variables influencing stereotactic accuracy and efficiency in deep brain stimulation surgery. Oper Neurosurg. 2019;17:70–8. https://doi.org/10.1093/ons/opy291.
13. Shao HM, Chen JY, Truong TK, Reed IS, Kwoh YS. A new CT-aided robotic stereotaxis system. Proc Annu Symp Comput Appl Med Care. 1985;13:668–72.
14. Kwoh YS, Hou J, Jonckheere EA, Hayati S. A robot with improved absolute positioning accuracy or CT guided stereotactic brain surgery. IEEE Trans Biomed Eng. 1988;35(2):153–60.
15. Haegelen C, Touzet G, Reyns N, et al. Stereotactic robot-guided biopsies of brain stem lesions: experience with 15 cases. Neurochirurgie. 2010;56(5):363–7.
16. Lefranc M, Touzet G, Caron S, et al. Are stereotactic sample biopsies still of value in the modern management of pineal region tumours? Lessons from a single-department, retrospective series. Acta Neurochir. 2011;153(5):1111–22.
17. Cossu M, Cardinale F, Castana L, et al. Stereoelectroencephalography in the presurgical evaluation of focal epilepsy: a retrospective analysis of 215 procedures. Neurosurgery. 2005;57(4):706–18.
18. Wu C, Jermakowicz WJ, Chakravorti S, Cajigas I, Sharan AD, Jagid JR, et al. Effects of surgical targeting in laser interstitial thermal therapy for mesial temporal lobe epilepsy: a multicenter study of 234 patients. Epilepsia. 2019;60:1171–83. https://doi.org/10.1111/epi.15565.
19. Lefranc M, Le Gars D. Robotic implantation of deep brain stimulation leads, assisted by intraoperative, flat-panel CT. Acta Neurochir. 2012 Nov;154(11):2069–74.
20. Lefranc M, Capel C, Pruvot-Ocean AS, Fichten A, Desenclos C, Toussaint P, et al. Frameless robotic stereotactic biopsies: a consecutive series of 100 cases. J Neurosurg. 2015;122(2):342–52.
21. Limousin P, Pollak P, Benazzouz A, Hoff-Mann D, Le Bas JF, Broussolle E, et al. Effect of parkinsonian signs and symptoms of bilateral subthalamic nucleus stimulation. Lancet. 1995;345(8942):91–5.

22. Ellis TM, Foote KD, Fernandez HH, Sudhyadhom A, Rodriguez RL, Zeilman P, et al. Reoperation for suboptimal outcomes after deep brain stimulation surgery. Neurosurgery. 2008 Oct;63(4):754–60.
23. Richardson RM, Ostrem JL, Starr PA. Surgical repositioning of misplaced subthalamic electrodes in Parkinson's disease: location of effective and ineffective leads. Stereotact Funct Neurosurg. 2009;87(5):297–303.
24. Steigerwald F, Müller L, Johannes S, Matthies C, Volkmann J. Directional deep brain stimulation of the subthalamic nucleus: a pilot study using a novel neurostimulation device. Mov Disord. 2016;31(8):1240–3.
25. Hariz MI. Complications of deep brain stimulation surgery. Mov Disord. 2002;17(S3):162–6.
26. Lefranc M, Capel C, Pruvot AS, Fichten A, Desenclos C, Toussaint P, et al. The impact of the reference imaging modality, registration method and intraoperative flat-panel computed tomography on the accuracy of the ROSA stereotactic robot. Stereotact Funct Neurosurg. 2014;92(4):242–50.
27. Li QH, Zamorano L, Pandya A, Perez R, Gong J, Diaz F. The application accuracy of the NeuroMate robot - a quantitative comparison with frameless and frame-based surgical localization systems. Comput Aided Surg. 2002;7(2):90–8.
28. Wiebe S, Blume WT, Girvin JP, Eliasziw M. A randomized, controlled trial of surgery for temporal-lobe epilepsy. N Engl J Med. 2001;345:311–8.
29. Engel JJ, Wiebe S, French J, et al. Practice parameter: temporal lobe and localized neocortical resections for epilepsy: report of the Quality Standards Subcommittee of the American Academy of Neurology, in association with the American Epilepsy Society and the American Association of Neurology. Neurology. 2003;60:538–47.
30. Engel JJ, McDermott MP, Wiebe S, et al. Early surgical therapy for drug-resistant temporal lobe epilepsy. JAMA. 2012;307:922–30.
31. Dwivedi R, Ramanujam B, Chandra S, et al. Surgery for drug resistant epilepsy in children. N Engl J Med. 2018;378:398–9.
32. Kilpatrick C, Cook M, Kaye A, Murphy M, Matkovic Z. Non-invasive investigations successfully select patients for temporal lobe surgery. J Neurol Neurosurg Psychiatry. 1997;63(3):327–33.
33. Diehl B, Lüders HO. Temporal lobe epilepsy: when are invasive recordings needed? Epilepsia. 2000;41(Suppl 3):S61–74.
34. Zumsteg D, Wieser HG. Presurgical evaluation: current role of invasive EEG. Epilepsia. 2000;41(Suppl 3):S55–60.
35. Cossu M, Lo Russo G, Francione S, et al. Epilepsy surgery in children: results and predictors of outcome on seizures. Epilepsia. 2008;49(1):65–72.
36. González-Martínez J, Bulacio J, Thompson S, et al. Technique, results, and complications related to robot-assisted stereoelectroencephalography. Neurosurgery. 2016;78(2):169–80. https://academic.oup.com/neurosurgery/article/78/2/169/2453610
37. Cardinale F, Cossu M, Castana L, Casaceli G, Schiariti MP, Miserocchi A, et al. Stereoelectroencephalography: surgical methodology, safety, and stereotactic application accuracy in 500 procedures. Neurosurgery. 2013;72(3):353–66.
38. Mullin JP, Shriver M, Alomar S, et al. Is SEEG safe? A systematic review and meta-analysis of stereo-electroencephalographyrelated complications. Epilepsia. 2016;57:386–401.
39. Drane DL, Loring DW, Voets NL, Price M, Ojemann JG, Willie JT, et al. Better object recognition and naming outcome with MRI-guided stereotactic laser amygdalohippocampotomy for temporal lobe epilepsy. Epilepsia. 2015;56:101–13. https://doi.org/10.1111/epi.12860.
40. Voets NL, Alvarez I, Qiu D, Leatherday C, Willie JT, Sotiropoulos S, et al. Mechanisms and risk factors contributing to visual field deficits following stereotactic laser amygdalohippocampotomy. Stereotact Funct Neurosurg. 2019;97:255–65. https://doi.org/10.1159/000502701.
41. Jermakowicz WJ, Wu C, Neal E, Cajigas I, D'Haese PF, Donahue DJ, et al. Clinically significant visual deficits after laser interstitial thermal therapy for mesiotemporal epilepsy. Stereotact Funct Neurosurg. 2019;97:347–55. https://doi.org/10.1159/000504856.

42. Pauliah M, Saxena V, Haris M, Husain N, Rathore RKS, Gupta RK. Improved T1-weighted dynamic contrast-enhanced MRI to probe microvascularity and heterogeneity of human glioma. Magn Reson Imag. 2007;25(9):1292–9.
43. Kunz M, Thon N, Eigenbrod S, et al. Hot spots in dynamic18FET- PET delineate malignant tumor parts within suspected WHO grade II gliomas. Neuro-Oncology. 2011;13(3):307–16.
44. Zanello M, Roux A, Senova S, Peeters S, Edjlali M, Tauziede-Espariat A, Dezamis E, Parraga E, Zah-Bi G, Harislur M, Oppenheim C, Sauvageon X, Chretien F, Devaux B, Varlet P, Pallud J. Robot-assisted stereotactic biopsies in 377 consecutive adult patients with supratentorial diffuse gliomas: diagnostic yield, safety, and postoperative outcomes. World Neurosurg. 2021 Apr;148:e301–13. https://doi.org/10.1016/j.wneu.2020.12.127.
45. Marcus HJ, Vakharia VN, Ourselin S, Duncan J, Tisdall M, Aquilina K. Robot-assisted stereotactic brain biopsy: systematic review and bibliometric analysis. Childs Nerv Syst. 2018;34(7):1299–309. https://doi.org/10.1007/s00381-018-3821-y.
46. Chen C, Lee I, Tatsui C, Elder T, Sloan AE. Laser interstitial thermotherapy (LITT) for the treatment of tumors of the brain and spine: a brief review. J Neuro-Oncol. 2021;151(3):429–42. https://doi.org/10.1007/s11060-020-03652-z.
47. Schieferdecker S, Hunsche S, El Majdoub F, Maarouf M. Robot-assisted stereotactic shunting as a novel treatment for pontine glioependymal cysts. J Neurol Surg A Cent Eur Neurosurg. 2021; https://doi.org/10.1055/s-0041-1726109.
48. Doddamani RS, Meena R, Sawarkar D, Singh P, Agrawal D, Singh M, Chandra PS. Robot-guided ventriculoperitoneal shunt in slit-like ventricles. Neurol India. 2021;69(2):446–50. https://doi.org/10.4103/0028-3886.314585.
49. Liu HG, Liu DF, Zhang K, Meng FG, Yang AC, Zhang JG. Clinical application of a neurosurgical robot in intracranial ommaya reservoir implantation. Front Neurorobot. 2021;26(15):638633. https://doi.org/10.3389/fnbot.2021.638633.
50. Barua NU, Hopkins K, Woolley M, O'Sullivan S, Harrison R, Edwards RJ, et al. A novel implantable catheter system with transcutaneous port for intermittent convection-enhanced delivery of carboplatin for recurrent glioblastoma. Drug Deliv. 2016;23(1):167–73.

Robotics in Neuroendoscopy

Alba Madoglio, Elena Roca, Fabio Tampalini,
Marco Maria Fontanella, and Francesco Doglietto

1 Introduction

Neuroendoscopic surgery is a growing field in neurosurgery [1] and possibly the main variety of minimally invasive neurosurgery [2].

The dawn of neuroendoscopy was characterized by the technical limitations of the available endoscopes, which were severely restricted in depth of field, optical quality, and illumination. Initially used by pioneers as a diagnostic approach to the

A. Madoglio
Neurosurgery Unit, Department of Neuroscience and Rehabilitation, University of Ferrara, Ferrara, Italy
e-mail: alba.madoglio@edu.unife.it

E. Roca
Neurosurgery, Head and Neck Department, Istituto Ospedaliero Fondazione Poliambulanza, Brescia, Italy

"Technology for Health" Ph.D. Program, University of Brescia, Brescia, Italy
e-mail: e.roca@unibs.it

F. Tampalini
Department of Information Engineering, University of Brescia, Brescia, Italy
e-mail: fabio.tampalini@unibs.it

M. M. Fontanella
Neurosurgery, Department of Medical and Surgical Specialties, Radiological Sciences and Public Health, University of Brescia, Brescia, Italy
e-mail: marco.fontanella@unibs.it

F. Doglietto (✉)
Neurosurgery, Department of Medical and Surgical Specialities, Radiological Sciences and Public Health, University of Brescia, Brescia, Italy

Fondazione Policlinico Universitario Agostino Gemelli IRCCS, Rome, Italy

Catholic University School of Medicine, Rome, Italy
e-mail: francesco.doglietto@unibs.it

M. M. Al-Salihi et al. (eds.), *Introduction to Robotics in Minimally Invasive Neurosurgery*, https://doi.org/10.1007/978-3-030-90862-1_4

ventricular system and for managing hydrocephalus, neuroendoscopy was largely abandoned for decades owing to those technical limitations [1]. This period of darkness continued until the 1970s. Interest in endoscopic third ventriculostomy (ETV) for treating obstructive hydrocephalus was then renewed thanks to the improved imaging capacities of the endoscopes [3].

Harold Hopkins and Karl Storz introduced critical innovations that allowed for structural and functional improvement of the endoscope: improvement of illumination, better definition of anatomical details because of high-definition optics, and wide viewing lenses that overcame the previous narrow viewing angles. Those technical advances allowed neurosurgeons to see in areas otherwise hidden from microsurgical vision (the so-called view around the corner) and provided a different perception of anatomy [4]. It then became possible to improve visualization while ensuring less tissue trauma than in traditional open surgery: this was the turning point in endoscopy applied to neurosurgery [1, 5].

Since then, the neuroendoscope has been used in treating not only triventricular hydrocephalus but also intraventricular tumors (biopsy, drainage, or resection), skull base tumors, craniosynostosis, intracranial cystic lesions, and rare subtypes of hydrocephalus [6]. Endoscopy can also be used to assist microsurgery in virtually any kind of neurosurgical procedure (endoscope-assisted microsurgery), particularly for aneurysms and tumors [7]. The diversity of these disorders indicates the vast potential of endoscopy in neurosurgery [6]. In dealing with this range of pathological conditions, neuroendoscopy has to be specifically adapted to the different procedures and lesions being addressed. Various types of endoscopes with corresponding instruments are, therefore, available [5].

During the past two decades, neuronavigation systems and image-guided surgery have been applied to provide neurosurgeons with real-time imaging during endoscopic procedures. With the combination of image-guided surgery and neuronavigation technology, neuroendoscopy has the potential to overcome the limitations of microsurgical visualization, while the ability to track the tip of the endoscope could decrease the level of invasiveness and increase the safety of endoscopic procedures.

With conventional neuroendoscopic techniques, e.g. freehand endoscopy, or with the use of mechanical or pneumatic endoscope-holding devices, the amount of movement of the endoscope within the brain depends on the experience and manual skill of the individual neurosurgeon. Physiological tremor, inadvertent movements, and loss of orientation could in principle be eliminated by a robotic endoscope holder. These potential advantages have led to the development of robotic systems to assist surgeons in performing complex endoscopic neurosurgical procedures [8, 9].

This chapter reviews the different fields of cranial neuroendoscopy and the preclinical robots that have been developed for it, and the clinical robotic solutions that have been applied to the field of endoscopic minimally invasive cranial surgery.

2 Fields of Application of Cranial Neuroendoscopy

Three fields of cranial neuroendoscopy have been developed: ventricular neuroendoscopy, endoscopic transnasal skull base surgery, and pure endoscopic or endoscope-assisted cranial neurosurgery [7].

2.1 Ventricular Neuroendoscopy

2.1.1 Hydrocephalus

Endoscopic third ventriculostomy (ETV) is the most widely used neuroendoscopic procedure for treating non-communicating obstructive hydrocephalus of various etiologies. The success rate is not 100%, as approximately 25–40% of patients require insertion of a shunt during the postoperative period [7, 10]. In addition to ETV for treating triventricular hydrocephalus, the ventriculoscope has been used to perform other surgical procedures and to address other forms of obstructive hydrocephalus (septum pellucidotomy, fenestration of loculated ventricles, and aqueductoplasty for treating aqueductal stenosis) [3, 6].

2.1.2 Cyst and Intraventricular Tumors

Ventricular endoscopic procedures include cyst fenestration, tumor biopsy, and tumor removal. Most patients with intraventricular cysts or tumors have concomitant hydrocephalus, which can be treated concurrently with ETV or septostomy [3, 11]. The first to use neuroendoscopy to perform a biopsy were Fukushima and colleagues [6]. This approach ensures direct and high-definition visualization of the abnormal tissue, exploiting a minimal access that can be optimized using neuronavigation [11]. Somji and colleagues [12] reported the results of a meta-analysis of 30 studies for a total of nearly 2100 neuroendoscopic biopsies: the diagnostic yield was 87.9% [13]. Although this was slightly lower than the yield from open biopsies, the neuroendoscopic procedure has significant advantages: 1. less invasiveness, morbidity and mortality; 2. during the same procedure, the associated obstructive hydrocephalus can be treated [12, 13].

2.1.3 Hypothalamic Hamartomas

Hypothalamic hamartomas are rare congenital non-neoplastic lesions associated with intractable epilepsy, precocious puberty, personality disorders, and cognitive problems that intensify over time. Removal or disconnection can lead to complete remission (60%) or improvement (90%) of the seizure disorder [11]. Stereotaxic navigation-assisted endoscopic resection is useful for removing these small, focal lesions, although a part of the hamartoma remains in some circumstances. In most cases, navigation assistance is recommended because the lateral and third ventricles are normal in size in these patients [3].

2.2 Endoscopic Transnasal Skull Base Surgery

The Austrian surgeons Messerklinger and Stammberger pioneered a revolutionary new procedure: they developed the concept of functional endoscopic sinus surgery [14], which evolved into endoscopic transsphenoidal surgery for treating sellar tumors and, more recently, into endoscopic transnasal skull base surgery (ESBS) [15].

2.2.1 Transsphenoidal Surgery in the Sellar Region

Endoscopic transsphenoidal surgery was developed during the late 1990s in Pittsburgh by Carrau and Jho, who reported the first surgical series, soon followed by studies from Cappabianca and De Divitiis in Naples, Frank and Pasquini in

Bologna, and other centers in Europe and North America [3]. Since then the technique has been further developed, thanks to new technological advances such as the development of high-definition optics.

2.2.2 Transnasal Skull Base Surgery

The close collaboration between ENT and neurosurgeons has led to the full development of endoscopic transnasal skull base surgery during the past two decades [3]. With the increasing complexity of transnasal endoscopic surgery, the need for a bimanual dissection has become evident [16] and the so-called four hands technique has been developed [17]. Operating times have also increased in parallel with the complexity of the procedures, which can address many different pathologies of the skull base [18, 19].

2.3 Neuroendoscopy-Assisted Cranial Microsurgery

Perneczky and Fries pioneered the concept of endoscope-assisted microsurgery: the endoscope can be the sole visualization tool or it can be coupled with the microscope in the so-called endoscope-assisted microneurosurgery [20, 21]. It combines the advantages of the surgical microscope with those of the endoscope such as improved illumination, definition of details, and a marked increase in viewing angles [7]. The operating microscope provides a stereoscopic view and displays the surface structures in high definition. However, there is a limited field of view in deep and narrow surgical corridors and light is lost at the entry site, so high-definition endoscopes with various angles of view are useful [7, 21]. The endoscope has indeed been reported as a useful complement to the microscope in anterior skull base surgery, posterior fossa approaches, and aneurysm surgery [3].

Endoscopic-assisted techniques have frequently been applied to cerebellopontine angle (CPA) surgery in the context of minimally invasive craniotomies. The advantages of the endoscope have been emphasized in minimally invasive surgery, reducing morbidity by minimizing soft tissue dissection. Abolfotoh et al. showed the advantages of using the endoscope in cerebellopontine angle surgery: (1) extension of the surgical field into further intracranial compartments and (2) visualization and resection of residual tumor not visualized under the microscope [22].

3 Robotics in Neuroendoscopy

Studies on robotics in neuroendoscopy were implemented, in particular, with the birth of minimally invasive surgery. The theoretical advantages of surgical robotics systems are greater precision, tremor filtration for improved image stability, and reduced fatigue for the surgical team, motion scaling, and bimanual manipulation.

Robotics systems can be classified into three categories on the basis of how surgeons interact with them (Fig. 1):

1. *Supervisory-controlled robot systems* in which the surgeon plans the operation and the robot then carries it out autonomously under the supervision of the surgeon (Fig. 1a);

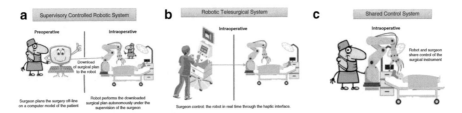

Fig. 1 Three categories of robotic systems according to user-interaction. (**a**) Supervisory controlled system; (**b**) Telesurgical system; (**c**) Shared control system

2. *Telesurgical (master-slave) systems* in which the surgeon (master) remotely controls the robot's actions (slave) (Fig. 1b);
3. *Handheld shared-controlled systems* in which the surgeon and robot share control of the instrument (Fig. 1c).

Although a multitude of robots have been applied to neurosurgery, few are applicable to minimally invasive techniques. Different robotics prototypes have been developed for neuroendoscopy, but only some of these have been applied clinically in preliminary studies [23] (Table 1).

3.1 Robotics in Intraventricular Procedures

3.1.1 Supervisory-Controlled Robot Systems

LightWeight robot (LWR) is a supervisory-controlled system that enables surgery to be image-guided. A handling interface for linking an endoscope to a seven DoF (Degrees of Freedom) lightweight robot (LWR) (tool holder), namely the LightWeight IV+ arm (Kuka Roboter), has been developed and tested in a preclinical model [31]. Niccolini and coworkers [31] investigated the accuracy of targeting in a ventriculostomy model in which the robot was operated both autonomously and in hands-on mode (i.e., cooperative). In most cases a satisfactory average accuracy was achieved; no significant differences were highlighted between the hands-on and autonomous control modes in the insertion/retraction movements. This supports the approach adopted, which combines both control modes. Surgeon feedback on the developed handling interface was positive, and so were the results of preliminary targeting tests, and Niccolini and coworkers [31] concluded that both sources of feedback fully supported further platform development and assessment. Furthermore, they emphasized that research should also concentrate on the development and validation of ETV tools.

3.1.2 Telesurgical (Master–Slave) Systems

Hongo and coworkers presented three studies on *NeuRobot* (Shinshu University School of Medicine, Matsumoto, Japan), the first telesurgical robot designed specifically for keyhole neurosurgery [25, 32, 33]. Their first study [32] described the micromanipulator system and presented the preliminary results of a cadaveric

Table 1 Preliminary clinical applications of robotic systems in neuroendoscopy

Robot name	Type of control	Features	Type of surgery (no. of patients enrolled)	Selected studies
Evolution 1 (Universal Robot Systems, Schwerin, Germany)	Shared control	– Hexapod robot with six DoF[a] – Endoscope holder – Joystick (TM)	ETV (six patients)	Zimmermann (2002–2004) [9, 24]
Neurobot (Shinshu, University School of Medicine, Matsumoto, Japan)	Telesurgical	– Nine DoF (three sets of micromanipulators, each with three DoF) – Rigid 3D endoscope	ETV (one patient)	Takasuna et al. (2012) [25]
–	–	– EEA-TORS approach: Ability to reach the posterior skull base below the level of the Eustachian tube with TORS – EEA phase not performed with the robot (limit of robotics)	EEA-TORS approach (two patients)	Carrau et al. (2013) [26]
ROSA (Medtech, Montepellier, France)	Supervisory controlled and shared control	– Image-guided device with six DoF – Offline integrated planning system	HH (20 patients)	Calisto et al. (2014) [27]
			ETV (five patients); HH disconnection (24 patients); septostomy (two patients); biopsy (eight patients)	De Benedictis et al. (2017) [28]
			ETV (nine patients)	Hoshide et al. (2017) [29]
i-ArmS (Denso robotics)	–	– Robotic arm rest – Three modes: transfer (Free), arm holding (Hold), and arm free (Wait)	ETSS (43 patients)	Ogiwara et al. (2017) [30]
Endoscope Robot® (Medineering Surgical Robots, Munich, Germany)	Shared control	– Hybrid robotic solution for ESBS with seven DoF – Endoscope holder – Foot pedal	ESBS (21 patients)	Zappa et al. (2021) [57]

ROSA robotized stereotactic assistant, *ETV* endoscopic third ventriculostomy, *HH* hypotalamic hamartoma, *ESBS* endoscopic skull base surgery, *EEA-TORS* endoscopic endonasal approach-transoral robotic surgery, *ETSS* endoscopic endonasal transsphenoidal surgery, *TM* telemanipulation mode, *DoF* degrees of freedom

[a]The "neuroendoscopy" software module used for these patients restricts the movement of the attached endoscope to four DoF

experimental study (simulating a third ventriculostomy). The complete system consists of four main parts: the micromanipulator (slave manipulator), the manipulator-supporting device, the operation-input device (master manipulator), and the 3D display monitor. It has a single-shaft design, which is approximately 10 mm in diameter and contains a 3-dimensional endoscope and three sets of micromanipulators, each with three DoF (rotation, neck swinging, and forward/backward motion) [23].

Hongo et al. [33] confirmed NeuRobot as suitable and safe for performing sophisticated surgical procedures less invasively, but they concluded that further developments were needed to improve its maneuverability, as also reported by Takasuna and coworkers [25]. Four different intraventricular procedures were simulated in three fixed cadaver heads and then carried out; a third ventriculostomy on a patient with obstructive hydrocephalus due to a midbrain venous angioma was performed safely. Although the system could perform relatively simple surgical procedures in cadaver and human studies, the authors concluded that the maneuverability of both the micromanipulators and the robot itself need to be improved before widespread clinical application is considered [23].

3.1.3 Shared Control Systems

In 2002, after preclinical anatomical and precision studies, Zimmermann et al. [24] presented their preliminary clinical experience with robot-assisted navigated neuroendoscopic procedures, and in 2004 they demonstrated their first clinical experience with the same robot in navigated endoscopic third ventriculostomies [9].

Evolution 1 (Universal Robot Systems, Schwerin, Germany) [9, 24, 34], a modular robotic teleoperation system controlled directly by the surgeon via a joystick and based on a Stewart platform (hexapod design) with a seven axis (z-axis), was tested in both studies. In their preliminary studies, the authors demonstrated the advantage of Evolution 1 as an endoscope holder and positioning device. This system allows for smooth slow movements in critical regions and can be stopped immediately, thus avoiding unwanted movements. It is safe, but limited by a range of motion of 30°, a limit that becomes evident if endoscopic procedures that require a larger range of motion are planned (e.g., ventriculostomy combined with fenestration of a cyst) [9, 24]. This robotic system was then modified for transsphenoidal endoscopic surgery (see the dedicated paragraph for further details) [34].

3.1.4 Continuum Robots

A different robotic concept was developed to access deep intracranial spaces such as the cerebral ventricles while eliminating the need to tilt the endoscope, which causes compression and injury to the brain tissue through which the endoscope passes [35]. These "continuum" or "snake-like" robotic systems include concentric tube robots and tendon-driven robots; they avoid traditional long and rigid connections in favor of flexible curving segments. They can provide the required dexterity without endoscope tilting while carrying surgical instruments in their inner lumina.

A concentric tube robot comprises several pre-curved concentric tubes differing in flexibility. Precise control relies on advanced kinematic models to account for a variety of phenomena including bending, torsion, nonlinear constitutive effects, friction, material hysteresis, and clearance [36]. Butler et al. [36] presented a concentric tube system associated with a robotically controlled flexible endoscope. The tendon-driven continuum robot developed and described in several studies by Kato and coworkers [2, 37] also belongs to this group of continuum robotic systems. Previous studies [38, 39] showed that the hysteresis in their tendon-driven robot could have resulted from the friction between tendons and robots and could cause errors in estimating the posture of tendon-driven devices [37].

Kato et al. [2, 37] introduced an extended forward kinematic mapping (FKM) with attention to the hysteresis operation of the robot. The extended FKM maps tension in tendons to the posture of the robot as time-discrete variables and amends the previous posture to the present one. In the experimental results, the extended FKM predicted the postures in the hysteresis operation with improved accuracy.

Rox et al. [35] described a two-arm concentric tube robot system. It is composed of robot, neuroendoscope, and concentric tube manipulators. The robot uses a compact differential drive and features embedded motor control electronics and redundant position sensors for safety. To highlight the characteristics of this system, the authors decided to simulate a colloid cyst resection surgical environment in a phantom based on a patient CT scan [35]. Qualitatively, the presence of a second, dexterous tool completely changed the surgical approach. In particular, the ability to apply tension and retraction and to use the arms cooperatively enabled the surgeon to perform more complex surgical maneuvers to manipulate the cyst without requiring endoscope angulation. Furthermore, by switching from a manual to a robotic procedure, the number of surgeons required was reduced from two to one. The authors concluded that future work should optimize the overlap between the workspace of the concentric tubes and the endoscope field of view.

A continuum robot controlled by FTL (follow-the-leader) motion planning was developed to perform a combined endoscopic third ventriculostomy (ETV) and endoscopic tumor biopsy (ETB) procedure [40].

Wang et al. [41] developed a novel continuum robotic sheath for neuroendoscopy in which the sheath is designed to provide two robotic arms. It is a two-channel eccentric-tube robot with two continuum arms delivered through the channels. Tube rotation at the proximal end controls the shape of the sheath and thus the direction of the work. Starting from this prototype, the authors proposed to extend the work by adding, for example, another arm that could be used for the imaging system; the three activation tubes would then match the standard number of push/pull tendons.

3.2   Robotics in Endoscopic Transnasal Skull Base Surgery

Several prototypes for endoscopic transnasal skull base surgery have been developed, but they have some disadvantages including ergonomics and prolonged set-up time [42, 43]. They can be classified into cooperative, continuum, and hybrid robotic systems.

3.2.1 Telemanipulation Mode and Cooperative Mode

These prototypes can be classified according to the type of interface they use: telemanipulation mode or "cooperative mode."

Only two of them are controlled in cooperative mode (i.e., surgeon and robotic arm cooperate side by side to hold the endoscope): [42] (1) an image-guided robot system described by Xia et al. [44] that includes a modified integrated navigation system (NeuroMate®, Integrated Surgical Systems, Sacramento, CA) and has the function of endoscope/drill-holder; (2) *HYBRID* [45], a hybrid solution that has the task of holding the endoscope, remaining entirely dependent on the surgeon, has a force threshold as an interface.

Most prototypes controlled in telemanipulation mode (e.g. voice control, head motion, foot pedal, and joystick) are joystick-controlled, though many authors have noted that this requires an additional surgeon who needs to be extremely well coordinated with the primary surgeon.

- Joystick control: (1) *Evolution 1* (EVO1) [34], modified for transsphenoidal endoscopic surgery since its first implementation for ventriculostomy (see earlier paragraph for further details). It has six DoF and an additional z-axis that increases the workspace; (2) *A-73* [46], an automatic robotic system based on a 3D navigation system and "loss of control" mode; (3) *Tx40* [47] has autonomous tracking movements and an automatic lens cleaning system; (4) the *Stewart Platform (SP)-based robotic system* [16] has a resistance felt on the haptic arm if there is contact or friction with adjacent tissues; (5) Strauß et al. [48] described a robotic system integrated with a navigation system in which it is easy to switch to the manual endoscopic system if necessary; (6) Yoon et al. [49] developed a double joystick to control the active bending of the endoscope prototype coupled with a spring backbone.
- Voice control: (1) the Automated Endoscopic System for Optimal Positioning (*AESOP*) robot [50] has the peculiarity of being able to memorize three positions to which the surgeon can return with a single voice command.
- Foot pedal control: (1) Foot-Controlled Robotic-Enabled Endoscope (*FREE*) [51] is controlled by an inertial measurement unit (IMU), the foot control interface, which is attached to the surgeon's foot and communicates with the control unit via Bluetooth. This set-up allows the foot's relative orientation to be measured in real time.

3.2.2 Continuum Robotic Systems

Continuum robotic systems have been described not only for intraventricular endoscopic surgery but also for ESBS [52, 53].

Swaney et al. [53] initially designed a novel 24 DoF quadramanual slave robot, controlled by the surgeon in console, and subsequently modified it [54] by adding the ability to rotate the end effector while leaving the robot fixed in space (i.e., ability to change the axial orientation of the angled ring curette without changing the tip position or orientation of the robot).

In the context of concentric tube robots, Wirz et al. [55] described the first remote telesurgery experiment (a phantom pituitary tumor removal experiment) in ESBS involving tentacle-like concentric tube manipulators. This led to the recent development of the first robot specifically designed for endonasal surgery. The prototype was similar to other continuum robots, but in this case the authors used the system to explore the idea of remotely controlling surgical tools over long distances for endonasal skull base surgery, the surgeon's commands being transmitted over the internet to a remote location.

3.2.3　Hybrid Robotic Systems

In addition to the hybrid system described by Bolzoni et al. [42] reported a hybrid prototype, Brescia Endoscope Assistant Robotic (*BEAR*) holder, developed and tested preclinically at the University of Brescia. It is defined as hybrid because the robotic system is not "pure": it has the task of holding the endoscope while remaining entirely dependent on the surgeon. BEAR uses head control (marked glasses) to control the movement of the robot-held endoscope. It has limitations—ergonomics, suboptimal joint movements, and excessive inertia—because the robot used to create the prototype was a commercially available one used in the industry.

3.2.4　Clinical Applications in ESBS

Clinical applications in ESBS are limited to a robotic arm rest [30], to transoral robotic surgery (TORS) combined with an extended endonasal approach (EEA-TORS) [26], and to a preliminary experience with a hybrid robotic solution [56].

I-ArmS [30] is an intelligent arm-support system. The system has three modes: transfer (Free), arm holding (Hold), and arm free (Wait). When the surgeon's arm is placed on the arm holder the mode changes from Wait to Hold. When the surgeon's arm moves to the desired position and holds still the mode changes from Free to Hold. The mode is changed from Hold to Free with a click action by the surgeon's arm. I-ArmsS was designed to prevent hand tremor and to alleviate fatigue during surgery. The main limit of the system is that it does not substitute the surgeon's arm but is indeed an armrest.

Carrau et al. [26] described an *EEA-TORS* approach that provided excellent exposure of the posterior skull base, nasopharynx, and infratemporal fossa. The main advantage of this technique for managing skull base tumors is the ability to reach the posterior skull base below the level of the Eustachian tube, which is the inferior limit of the EEA, using TORS. This study, by an extremely experienced group, confirms the current limits of robotics as the EEA phase was not performed with the robot.

Recently, a hybrid robotic solution for ESBS has become available for clinical practice (*Endoscope Robot®*, Medineering, Munich, Germany) (Figs. 2, 3, and 4). It is a compact robot specifically developed to work as an endoscope holder during transnasal interventions and is made of a robotic arm together with a smaller robot that acts as an endoscope holder and can be controlled with a foot pedal. The positioning arm has seven DoF so it can be driven in every position of space by the simultaneous manual unlocking of two joints. Its superior end is connected to the

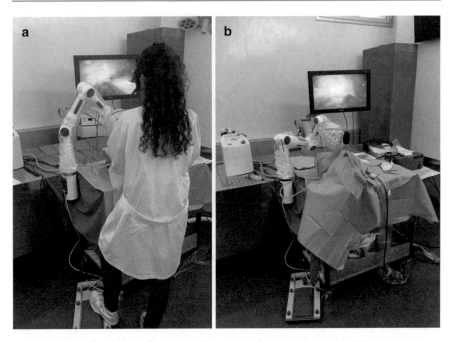

Fig. 2 Endoscope Robot® (Medineering, Munich, Germany). (**a**, **b**) Laboratory set-up at the University of Brescia

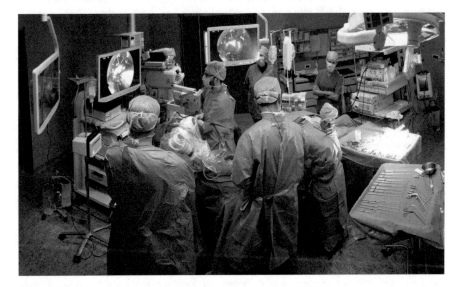

Fig. 3 Overview of the operating room during a robotic endoscopic transnasal skull base surgery at the University of Brescia

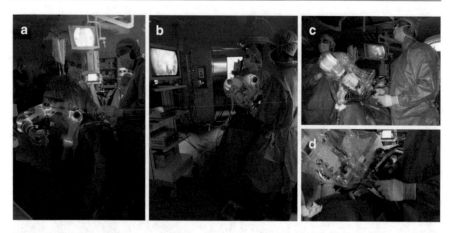

Fig. 4 Endoscope Robot® in the operating room at the University of Brescia. (**a**) During the nasal phase of surgery, the robot is away from the surgical field. (**b–d**) During the neurosurgical phase, the endoscope is held by Endoscope Robot® and positioned inside the nasal cavity. It can be orientated upwards, downwards or laterally using the joystick on the foot pedal; furthermore, it can be moved in or out by pressing different pads on the foot pedal. Foot pedal buttons can be used to save positions so the robot can automatically reposition the endoscope

endoscope holder. Once attached to the holder and positioned inside the nasal cavity, the endoscope can be oriented upwards, downwards or laterally using the joystick on the foot pedal. Furthermore, it can be moved in or out by pressing different pads on the foot pedal. Also, one particular button has the function of making the robot return to a previously saved "home position" at any moment during surgery. Zappa et al. [56] provided a preclinical evaluation of the potential advantages and surgeons' first impressions of a hybrid robotic solution for ESBS. Endoscope Robot seems to provide a benefit to the single surgeon with experience in bimanual endoscopic surgery. The same group then described the first clinical series of robotic endoscopic transnasal surgery, providing a clinical evaluation of potential advantages of this novel hybrid solution and the surgeons' subjective impressions [57].

3.3 Robotics in Minimally Invasive Endoscopic Pediatric Neurosurgery

Robotic-assisted surgery is of particular interest in pediatric neurosurgery. Developing structures are more vulnerable than the developed structures in adults, especially for small and deep targets. Furthermore, the normal anatomy of a child's brain is often altered by congenital malformations or by the disease itself, so neurosurgical management requires a high degree of intraoperative precision to identify and reach the surgical target without injuring the surrounding neurovascular structures [28].

Bodani et al. [58] developed a miniaturized, teleoperated, three-DoF concentric tube robot for pediatric intraventricular neuroendoscopy. In their report the authors presented both the design of the robot and its ability to perform an ETV in a phantom hydrocephalus brain model. Concentric tube continuum robots consist of telescopic, pre-curved, and superelastic tubes. The precision, dexterity, and reachability of the instrument added to this prototype were sufficient to perform an ETV successfully and have the potential to overcome the limitations of standard neuroendoscopic techniques [58].

In the literature, some authors have reported the clinical use of the *Robotized Stereotactic Assistant* (*ROSA*, Medtech) in pediatric neurosurgery. The ROSA system is a recently developed image-guided device that provides guidance for spatial positioning and orientation of several neurosurgical instruments according to a planned trajectory. According to the classification by Nathoo et al. [59], ROSA belongs to both categories of supervisory-controlled and shared-controlled systems. In this modality, the surgeon, after offline planning, can either supervise the robot performing the motion autonomously or directly control and move the surgical instrument during the procedure.

De Benedictis et al. [28] reported the results of a study of 116 pediatric patients who underwent surgical procedures for various pathologies with the assistance of the ROSA system. They performed 42 endoscopic procedures under ROSA guidance for managing different diseases, i.e. secondary obstructive hydrocephalus (seven cases), arachnoid cyst (three cases), intraventricular tumors (eight cases), and HHs (24 cases). The aim of the study was to validate this robotic assistance technique first in easier cases and later in more complex cases, as pediatric patients have a high incidence of hydrocephalus-related diseases, a narrow ventricular system, and deeply localized lesions. In all these cases, the robotic system guided the endoscope to the planned target. For HHs, the robot was useful for accessing the lateral ventricle safely and easily guiding the disconnection and coagulation laser. The results of the study showed the versatility of ROSA, given the possibility of integrating different tools. More studies are needed to validate previous results and improve current technology.

A previous study reported a preliminary analysis of results on the use of a thulium laser applied through robot-assisted endoscopy to disconnection surgery for HHs in a group of 20 pediatric patients. ROSA, a robotic neuronavigation system, was used to control the endoscope, allowing the ventriculostomy to be performed with millimetric precision, with limited movement along a predetermined trajectory or a "safe" space [27].

Hoshide et al. [29] used the ROSA robotic system to perform the ETVs procedure on nine pediatric patients. In accordance with other authors [27, 28], they reported the system to be stable, precise, and minimally invasive; in addition, the surgeon's learning curve was improved, with successive shortening of operating times.

Another clinical application of the robotic-assisted endoscopic approach has been in epilepsy surgery [60, 61], especially in children with drug-resistant epilepsy arising from hemispheric diseases. The hemispherotomy is performed by a hemispheric approach via a small pre-coronal craniotomy using an endoscope attached to a robotic arm (Rosa, Zimmer Biomet, Westminster, CO).

The benefits of robotic systems combined with endoscopes, i.e. stability, easy maneuverability in critical areas, and integrated navigation, lie in providing minimally invasive, safe, and effective surgery [25, 62]. It is clear that future studies will be needed to improve the adoption of this new technology.

4   Conclusion and Future Perspectives

Different prototypes have been produced for neuroendoscopy, but they have some limitations including bulky dimensions, poor ergonomics, inefficient control, and limited precision. To improve the present results, multidisciplinary collaboration is required, with novel solutions in terms of robot-control and specific instrumentation to exploit the advantages of endoscope robotic systems fully.

The need for collaborations with other sectors, in particular engineering, is evident: the development of new materials could allow the brain to be dynamically retracted, which would be necessary to develop the concept of transcranial, robot-assisted endoscope-microneurosurgery fully.

Another interesting area of research is represented by training in neurosurgical robotics. Comparative studies that assess resident training using traditional methods vs. robotics will be essential for determining the benefits of robotic surgery in neurosurgery; furthermore, they will be of paramount importance for optimizing training and fully exploiting the theoretical advantages of robotic surgery.

References

1. Zacharia BE, Schwartz TH. Diffusion of Neuroendoscopy: guided by the light. World Neurosurg. 2015;83(5):752–3. https://doi.org/10.1016/j.wneu.2014.10.010.
2. Kato T, Okumura I, Kose H, Takagi K, Hata N. Extended kinematic mapping of tendon-driven continuum robot for neuroendoscopy. In: 2014 IEEE/RSJ international conference on intelligent robots and systems. IEEE; 2014:1997–2002. https://doi.org/10.1109/IROS.2014.6942828.
3. Shim KW. Neuroendoscopy : current and future perspectives. Published online 2017:5.
4. Perneczky A, Tschabitscher M, Resch KDM. Endoscopic anatomy for neurosurgery. G. Thieme Verlag; 1993.
5. Esposito F, Cappabianca P. Neuroendoscopy: general aspects and principles. World Neurosurg. 2013;79(2):S14.e7–9. https://doi.org/10.1016/j.wneu.2012.02.033.
6. Li KW, Nelson C, Suk I, Jallo GI. Neuroendoscopy: past, present, and future. Neurosurg Focus. 2005;19(6):1–5. https://doi.org/10.3171/foc.2005.19.6.2.
7. Cinalli G, Cappabianca P, de Falco R, et al. Current state and future development of intracranial neuroendoscopic surgery. Expert Rev Med Devices. 2005;2(3):351–73. https://doi.org/10.1586/17434440.2.3.351.
8. Di Ieva A, Tam M, Tschabitscher M, Cusimano MD. A journey into the technical evolution of neuroendoscopy. World Neurosurg. 2014;82(6):e777–89. https://doi.org/10.1016/j.wneu.2014.09.005.
9. Zimmermann M, Krishnan R, Raabe A, Seifert V. Robot-assisted navigated endoscopic ventriculostomy: implementation of a new technology and first clinical results. Acta Neurochir. 2004;146(7) https://doi.org/10.1007/s00701-004-0267-7.
10. Enchev Y, Oi S. Historical trends of neuroendoscopic surgical techniques in the treatment of hydrocephalus. Neurosurg Rev. 2008;31(3):249–62. https://doi.org/10.1007/s10143-008-0131-y.

11. Cappabianca P, Cinalli G, Gangemi M, et al. Application of neuroendoscopy to intraventricular lesions. Neurosurgery. 2008;62(Suppl_2):SHC575–98. https://doi.org/10.1227/01. neu.0000316262.74843.dd.

12. Somji M, Badhiwala J, McLellan A, Kulkarni AV. Diagnostic yield, morbidity, and mortality of intraventricular neuroendoscopic biopsy: systematic review and meta-analysis. World Neurosurg. 2016;85:315–324.e2. https://doi.org/10.1016/j.wneu.2015.09.011.

13. Goldstein HE, Anderson RCE. The era of neuroendoscopy: just how far can we go? World Neurosurg. 2016;87:656–8. https://doi.org/10.1016/j.wneu.2015.10.046.

14. Trévillot V, Garrel R, Dombre E, Poignet P, Sobral R, Crampette L. Robotic endoscopic sinus and skull base surgery: review of the literature and future prospects. Eur Ann Otorhinolaryngol Head Neck Dis. 2013;130(4):201–7. https://doi.org/10.1016/j.anorl.2012.03.010.

15. Doglietto F, Prevedello DM, Jane JA, Han J, Laws ER. A brief history of endoscopic transsphenoidal surgery—from Philipp Bozzini to the First World Congress of Endoscopic Skull Base Surgery. Neurosurg Focus. 2005;19(6):1–6. https://doi.org/10.3171/foc.2005.19.6.4.

16. Cabuk B, Ceylan S, Anik I, Tugasaygi M, Kizir S. A haptic guided robotic system for endoscope positioning and holding. Turk Neurosurg. 2014; https://doi.org/10.5137/1019-5149. JTN.13290-14.0.

17. Castelnuovo P, Pistochini A, Locatelli D. Different surgical approaches to the sellar region: focusing on the "Two Nostrils Four Hands Technique". Rhinology. 2006;44(1):2–7.

18. Marciano F, Mattogno PP, Codenotti A, Cocca P, Fontanella MM, Doglietto F. Work-related musculoskeletal disorders among endoscopic transsphenoidal surgeons: a systematic review of prevalence and ergonomic interventions. Int J Occup Saf Ergon JOSE. 2020;1:1–10. https://doi.org/10.1080/10803548.2020.1774160.

19. Mattogno PP, Marciano F, Catalino MP, et al. Ergonomics in endoscopic trans-sphenoidal surgery: a survey of the North American Skull Base Society. J Neurol Surg Part B Skull Base. 2021; https://doi.org/10.1055/s-0041-1729906.

20. Schroeder HWS, Oertel J, Gaab MR. Endoscope-assisted microsurgical resection of epidermoid tumors of the cerebellopontine angle. J Neurosurg. 2004;101(2):227–32. https://doi.org/10.3171/jns.2004.101.2.0227.

21. Schroeder HWS. Transcranial endoscope-assisted skull base surgery – posterior fossa. Innov Neurosurg. 2013;1(1) https://doi.org/10.1515/ins-2012-0009.

22. Abolfotoh M, Bi WL, Hong C-K, et al. The combined microscopic-endoscopic technique for radical resection of cerebellopontine angle tumors. J Neurosurg. 2015;123(5):1301–11. https://doi.org/10.3171/2014.10.JNS141465.

23. Marcus HJ, Seneci CA, Payne CJ, Nandi D, Darzi A, Yang G-Z. Robotics in keyhole transcranial endoscope-assisted microsurgery: a critical review of existing systems and proposed specifications for new robotic platforms. Oper Neurosurg. 2014;10(1):84–96. https://doi.org/10.1227/NEU.0000000000000123.

24. Zimmermann M. Robot-assisted navigated neuroendoscopy. Published online 2002:7.

25. Takasuna H, Goto T, Kakizawa Y, et al. Use of a micromanipulator system (NeuRobot) in endoscopic neurosurgery. J Clin Neurosci. 2012;19(11):1553–7. https://doi.org/10.1016/j.jocn.2012.01.033.

26. Carrau RL, Prevedello DM, de Lara D, Durmus K, Ozer E. Combined transoral robotic surgery and endoscopic endonasal approach for the resection of extensive malignancies of the skull base: combined TORS and EEA for Resection of Extensive Malignancies of Skull Base. Head Neck. 2013;35(11):E351–8. https://doi.org/10.1002/hed.23238.

27. Calisto A, Bulteau C, Delalande O. Endoscopic disconnection of hypothalamic hamartomas: safety and feasibility of robot-assisted, thulium laser–based procedures. J Neurosurg. 2014;14:10.

28. De Benedictis A, Trezza A, Carai A, et al. Robot-assisted procedures in pediatric neurosurgery. Neurosurg Focus. 2017;42(5):E7. https://doi.org/10.3171/2017.2.FOCUS16579.

29. Hoshide R, Calayag M, Meltzer H, Levy ML, Gonda D. Robot-assisted endoscopic third ventriculostomy: institutional experience in 9 patients. J Neurosurg Pediatr. 2017;20(2):125–33. https://doi.org/10.3171/2017.3.PEDS16636.

30. Ogiwara T, Goto T, Nagm A, Hongo K. Endoscopic endonasal transsphenoidal surgery using the iArmS operation support robot: initial experience in 43 patients. Neurosurg Focus. 2017;42(5):E10. https://doi.org/10.3171/2017.3.FOCUS16498.
31. Niccolini M, Castelli V, Diversi C, Kang B, Mussa F, Sinibaldi E. Development and preliminary assessment of a robotic platform for neuroendoscopy based on a lightweight robot: robotic platform for neuroendoscopy with a lightweight robot. Int J Med Robot. 2016;12(1):4–17. https://doi.org/10.1002/rcs.1638.
32. Hongo K, Kobayashi S, Kakizawa Y, et al. NeuRobot: telecontrolled micromanipulator system for minimally invasive microneurosurgery. Prelimin Results. 2002;51:985–8.
33. Hongo K, Goto T, Miyahara T, Kakizawa Y, Koyama J, Tanaka Y. Telecontrolled micromanipulator system (NeuRobot) for minimally invasive neurosurgery. In: Nimsky C, Fahlbusch R, editors. Medical technologies in neurosurgery, vol. 98. Vienna: Springer; 2006. p. 63–6. https://doi.org/10.1007/978-3-211-33303-7_9.
34. Nimsky CH, Rachinger J, Fahlbusch R. Adaptation of a hexapod-based robotic system for extended endoscope-assisted transsphenoidal skull base surgery. Min - Minim Invasive Neurosurg. 2004;47(1):41–6. https://doi.org/10.1055/s-2003-812465.
35. Rox MF, Ropella DS, Hendrick RJ, et al. Mechatronic design of a two-arm concentric tube robot system for rigid neuroendoscopy. IEEEASME Trans Mechatron. 2020;25(3):1432–43. https://doi.org/10.1109/TMECH.2020.2976897.
36. Butler EJ, Hammond-Oakley R, Chawarski S, et al. Robotic neuro-endoscope with concentric tube augmentation. Published online 2013:21.
37. Kato T, Okumura I, Kose H, Takagi K, Hata N. Tendon-driven continuum robot for neuro-endoscopy: validation of extended kinematic mapping for hysteresis operation. Int J Comput Assist Radiol Surg. 2016;11(4):589–602. https://doi.org/10.1007/s11548-015-1310-2.
38. Camarillo DB, Milne CF, Carlson CR, Zinn MR, Salisbury JK. Mechanics modeling of tendon-driven continuum manipulators. IEEE Trans Robot. 2008;24(6):1262–73. https://doi.org/10.1109/TRO.2008.2002311.
39. Kato T, Okumura I, Song S-E, Hata N. Multi-section continuum robot for endoscopic surgical clipping of intracranial aneurysms. In: Salinesi C, Norrie MC, Pastor Ó, editors. Advanced information systems engineering, vol. 7908. Berlin Heidelberg: Springer; 2013. p. 364–71. https://doi.org/10.1007/978-3-642-40811-3_46.
40. Gao Y, Takagi K, Kato T, Shono N, Hata N. Continuum robot with follow-the-leader motion for endoscopic third ventriculostomy and tumor biopsy. IEEE Trans Biomed Eng. 2020;67(2):379–90. https://doi.org/10.1109/TBME.2019.2913752.
41. Wang J, Ha J, Dupont PE. Steering a multi-armed robotic sheath using eccentric precurved tubes. In: 2019 international conference on robotics and automation (ICRA). IEEE; 2019. p. 9834–40. https://doi.org/10.1109/ICRA.2019.8794245.
42. Bolzoni Villaret A, Doglietto F, Carobbio A, Schreiber A. Robotic transnasal endoscopic skull base surgery: systematic review of the literature and report of a novel prototype for a hybrid system (BEAR). World Neurosurg. 2017:33.
43. Madoglio A, Zappa F, Mattavelli D, et al. Robotics in endoscopic transnasal skull base surgery: literature review and personal experience. In: Control systems design of bio-robotics and bio-mechatronics with advanced applications. Elsevier; 2020. p. 221–44. https://doi.org/10.1016/B978-0-12-817463-0.00008-3.
44. Xia T, Baird C, Jallo G, et al. An integrated system for planning, navigation and robotic assistance for skull base surgery: integrated system for skull base robotic surgery. Int J Med Robot. 2008;4(4):321–30. https://doi.org/10.1002/rcs.213.
45. Trévillot V, Sobral R, Dombre E, Poignet P, Herman B, Crampette L. Innovative endoscopic sino-nasal and anterior skull base robotics. Int J Comput Assist Radiol Surg. 2013;8(6):977–87. https://doi.org/10.1007/s11548-013-0839-1.
46. Wurm J, Dannenmann T, Bohr C, Iro H, Bumm K. Increased safety in robotic paranasal sinus and skull base surgery with redundant navigation and automated registration. Int J Med Robot. 2005;1(3):42–8. https://doi.org/10.1002/rcs.26.

47. Eichhorn KW, Bootz F. Clinical requirements and possible applications of robot assisted endoscopy in skull base and sinus surgery. Acta Neurochir. 2011;109:237–40.
48. Strauß G, Hofer M, Kehrt S, et al. Ein Konzept für eine automatisierte Endoskopführung für die Nasennebenhöhlenchirurgie. HNO. 2007;55(3):177–84. https://doi.org/10.1007/s00106-006-1434-3.
49. Yoon HS, Oh SM, Jeong JH. Active bending endoscope robot system for navigation through sinus area. IEEE/RSJ; 2011.
50. Nathan C-A, Chakradeo V, Malhotra K, D'Agostino H, Patwardhan R. The voice-controlled robotic assist scope holder AESOP for the endoscopic approach to the sella. Skull Base. 2006;16(03):123–31. https://doi.org/10.1055/s-2006-939679.
51. Chan JYK, Leung I, Navarro-Alarcon D, et al. Foot-controlled robotic-enabled endoscope holder for endoscopic sinus surgery: a cadaveric feasibility study: foot controlled robotic endoscope. Laryngoscope. 2016;126(3):566–9. https://doi.org/10.1002/lary.25634.
52. Schneider JS, Burgner J, Iii RJW, Iii PTR. Robotic surgery for the sinuses and skull base: what are the possibilities and what are the obstacles? Published online 2014:12.
53. Swaney PJ, Croom JM, Burgner J, et al. Design of a quadramanual robot for single-nostril skull base surgery. In: Volume 3: renewable energy systems; robotics; robust control; single track vehicle dynamics and control; stochastic models, control and algorithms in robotics; structure dynamics and smart structures. ASME; 2012. p. 387–93. https://doi.org/10.1115/DSCC2012-MOVIC2012-8536.
54. Swaney P, Gilbert H, Webster R, Russell P, Weaver K. Endonasal skull base tumor removal using concentric tube continuum robots: a phantom study. J Neurol Surg Part B Skull Base. 2014;76(02):145–9. https://doi.org/10.1055/s-0034-1390401.
55. Wirz R, Torres LG, Swaney PJ, et al. An experimental feasibility study on robotic endonasal tele-surgery. Neurosurgery. 2015;76(4):479–84. https://doi.org/10.1227/NEU.0000000000000623.
56. Zappa F, Mattavelli D, Madoglio A, et al. Hybrid robotics for endoscopic skull base surgery: preclinical evaluation and surgeon first impression. World Neurosurg. 2020;134:e572–80. https://doi.org/10.1016/j.wneu.2019.10.142.
57. Zappa F, Madoglio A, Ferrari M, et al. Hybrid robotics for endoscopic transnasal skull base surgery: single-Centre case series. Oper Neurosurg Hagerstown Md. 2021;21(6):426–35.
58. Bodani V, Azimian H, Looi T, Drake JM. Design and evaluation of a concentric tube robot for minimally- invasive endoscopic paediatric. Neurosurgery. 2014;61(Suppl 1):192.
59. Nathoo N, Çavuşoğlu MC, Vogelbaum MA, Barnett GH. In touch with robotics: neurosurgery for the future. Neurosurgery. 2005;56(3):421–33. https://doi.org/10.1227/01.NEU.0000153929.68024.CF.
60. Chandra PS, Kurwale N, Garg A, Dwivedi R, Malviya SV, Tripathi M. Endoscopy-assisted interhemispheric transcallosal hemispherotomy. Neurosurgery. 2015;76(4):485–95. https://doi.org/10.1227/NEU.0000000000000675.
61. Chandra PS, Subianto H, Bajaj J, et al. Endoscope-assisted (with robotic guidance and using a hybrid technique) interhemispheric transcallosal hemispherotomy: a comparative study with open hemispherotomy to evaluate efficacy, complications, and outcome. J Neurosurg Pediatr. 2019;23(2):187–97. https://doi.org/10.3171/2018.8.PEDS18131.
62. Chumnanvej S, Pillai BM, Chalongwongse S, Suthakorn J. Endonasal endoscopic transsphenoidal approach robot prototype: a cadaveric trial. Asian J Surg. 2021;44(1):345–51. https://doi.org/10.1016/j.asjsur.2020.08.011.

Robotics in Spinal Surgery

Darius Ansari and Ankit I. Mehta

1 Overview

The role of robotic assistance in spine surgery can be roughly categorized by the ways in which it is used: (1) control systems in which the machine is provided with instructions for predetermined actions that are then carried out with close surgeon supervision; (2) telesurgical systems that allow the surgeon to control robotic movements completely from a remote command; and (3) shared models in which the surgeon and robot simultaneously control commands [1]. Similarly, the impact of robotic assistance on several aspects of spine surgery can be considered: physical fatigue, operative length, and other characteristics, radiation exposure, accuracy of screw placement, patient outcomes, technical issues, and other outcomes, some of which are briefly overviewed below and explored in greater detail throughout this chapter.

Spine surgery requires precise motor skills to excise and manipulate bone and other connective tissue along with fine accuracy in manipulating the neural and vascular structures within, often while using small operative corridors. Injury to any of these structures entails the risk of neurological deficits or hemorrhage during either hardware placement or surgical exposure [2]. This is especially relevant in cases of deformity, trauma, or malignancy, where local anatomy can be distorted and consequently more complex and the use of surgical aides such as navigation and/or robotics can be of greater benefit to the surgeon. Additionally, robotic systems can allow the surgical team to access three-dimensional visualizations of the patient's anatomical layout and permits others to view the procedure remotely via telemetry [3]. For these reasons, the advent of intraoperative imaging and

D. Ansari (✉) · A. I. Mehta
Department of Neurosurgery, University of Illinois at Chicago, Chicago, IL, USA
e-mail: dansari2@uic.edu; ankitm@uic.edu

© The Author(s), under exclusive license to Springer Nature Switzerland AG 2022
M. M. Al-Salihi et al. (eds.), *Introduction to Robotics in Minimally Invasive Neurosurgery*, https://doi.org/10.1007/978-3-030-90862-1_5

navigation systems to be used in tandem with robotic surgical systems is desirable not only to optimize visualization and mechanical accuracy, but also to maintain the reproducibility of such standards of accuracy in the face of lengthy and strenuous procedures.

Robotic navigation in spinal surgery is also beneficial in terms of screw placement accuracy, as evidenced radiologically [4, 5]. Several studies have demonstrated lower rates of screw malposition using surgical robotics than by free-hand placement [6, 7]. While these benefits of radiological accuracy must be considered separately from clinical outcomes, such as readmission, reoperation, and other complications, robotic assistance can also be desirable for eliminating physiological hand tremors, especially in cases with small pedicle diameter or distorted anatomy [6]. Much less clear is the effect of robotic spinal surgery and navigation on clinical outcomes. Most studies to date have failed to demonstrate any positive effect of robotic spinal surgery on hospital length of stay, surgical site infections, major complications, or total complication rates [8, 9].

As with all applications of technology, a learning curve associated with the use of robotics in spine surgery is to be expected. It has been noted in the literature that earlier adoption of navigation in spine surgery has been associated with higher rates of complications such as pedicle breach [1]. Other studies have demonstrated a positive correlation between surgeon familiarity with the robot and accuracy of screw placement [10]. This effect should be considered in both the interpretation of scientific studies regarding robotics in spinal surgery and the personal adoption of the technology.

2   Devices

2.1   Mazor: SpineAssist

In 2004, the SpineAssist® (Mazor Robotics Ltd., Caesarea, Israel) became the first robot approved by the FDA specifically for the use in spine surgery (Table 1) [11]. The SpineAssist is a shared-control robot that can automatically move its arm along a predetermined path, as opposed to requiring the surgeon to follow (manually) a trajectory predetermined by navigation. After positioning for screw placement is established by the SpineAssist, the surgeon then performs all the drilling.

Table 1 Currently available surgical robotic systems

Manufacturer	System	Initial FDA approval
Intuitive surgical	da Vinci Surgical System®	2000 (for general laparoscopic procedures)
Mazor	SpineAssist®	2004
Mazor	Renaissance®	2011
Zimmer Biomet	ROSA®	2012
Mazor	Mazor X®	2016
Globus medical	Excelsius GPS®	2017

Spinal fusions using the SpineAssist are usually performed in five main steps, detailed here as adapted from D'Souza et al. [4] First, 1-mm preoperative CT scans of the spinal levels of interest are obtained, and the surgeon uses the software package of the robot to generate the desired screw trajectory. Thereafter, the SpineAssist uses the trajectories entered to calculate optimal screw sizes and coordinates; these data are stored within the robot. The trajectories can be modified if previously unavailable CT scans are obtained or if a preplanned trajectory requires modification, for example, at the surgeon's discretion intraoperatively. Second, the patient is placed in prone position on the operating table, and a mounting frame is attached to him/her to permit image registration for the robot [4]. Several options for mounting are available, and the position is selected after the anticipated characteristics of the operation have been considered, such as open versus percutaneous approach. Most frequently, the platform is attached to the patient's spinous processes using one Kirschner-wire (K-wire) and secured bilaterally to the patient with two additional K-wires. In minimally invasive approaches, the robot is attached to a frame that is propped up by percutaneously placed guide wires [4]. Other, less common approaches exist, such as securing the platform to a cranial process. Third, after the frame is secured, six fluoroscopic images are collected and synchronized with the preoperative images. Synchronization of different types of images in this manner permits the user to deploy intraoperative fluoroscopy with preoperative CT scans, if desired, and allows the robot to construct a map of the operational field and the surrounding anatomical structures [12]. Fourth, after the robot has been attached to the mounting frame, the robot arm is aligned automatically and verifies the planned trajectories. Fifth, a cannulated dilator, drill guide, and guidewire are placed through the robotic surgical arm and screws are placed using the guide wires. After the screws are placed, the robot is disassembled.

The popularity of the SpineAssist in clinical practice has led not only to its wide adoption but also to relatively detailed understanding of its main pitfalls [13]. Placement of screws can be complicated by malposition of the cannula, commonly along the lateral aspect of the spinous process. Sliding of the cannula along the screw entrance point can lead to screw positioning that is more lateral than determined preoperatively [4]. Additionally, instability of the frame can lead to dissociation between the machine positioning relative to the patient, ultimately distorting the anatomical map and thus the predetermined trajectory.

2.2   Mazor: Renaissance and Mazor X

Mazor's second-generation robot for spine surgery, the Renaissance® (Fig. 1), replaced the SpineAssist in 2011. The primary updates from its predecessor included improved image recognition algorithms and the option for the surgeon to flatten the bone manually around screw entry points prior to drilling [14]. The latter is intended to address the issues of cannula skidding along the bone, which can be excessively sloped, especially in cases of distorted/degenerated anatomy; though it is not immune to such errors [13].

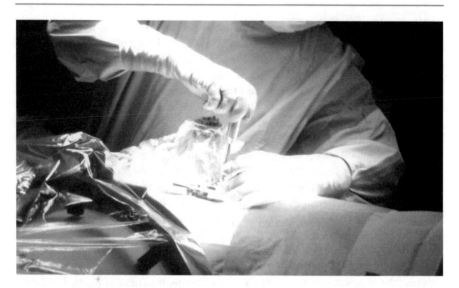

Fig. 1 Screw implantation following assistance with Renaissance® robotic system for posterior fusion. Image adapted from https://commons.wikimedia.org/wiki/File:Robotic_Spinal_Surgery.jpg, shared under GNU Free Documentation License. Accessed November 22, 2020

The most recent release by Mazor is the Mazor X®, introduced in 2016. Unlike its predecessors, the Mazor X features an integrated linear optic camera that enables it to self-detect its location and provide collision avoidance intraoperatively by performing 3D scans following reference placement [4]. It also includes a serial (rather than parallel) robotic arm that allows for increased range of motion and decreased reliance on surgical tools [15].

2.3   ROSA: SPINE

The ROSA® SPINE robot (Zimmer Biomet Robotics, Montpellier, France) was introduced in 2016 as a successor to its previous model for cranial operations [1]. The ROSA, similar to the aforementioned Mazor models, requires a preoperative CT scan; images captured from an O-arm® device within the operating room are automatically registered by the ROSA and a 3D reconstruction is generated. The surgeon can then merge the preoperative with intraoperative scans to plan the screw trajectory [16]. Intraoperative use of the ROSA is similar to that of the Mazor models: a guide tube needle is placed to facilitate guidewire threading on the posterior aspect of a target vertebral body, which the surgeon later uses to thread a cannulated dilator and insert screws under real-time navigation [3]. The major advantage of the ROSA is this real-time guidance feature performed on the basis of the 3D mapping generated at the beginning of the procedure [4]. Like other robots, the ROSA is limited by a lengthy setup and the inability to move the patient or camera, as this would result in inaccurate mapping and screw placement [17].

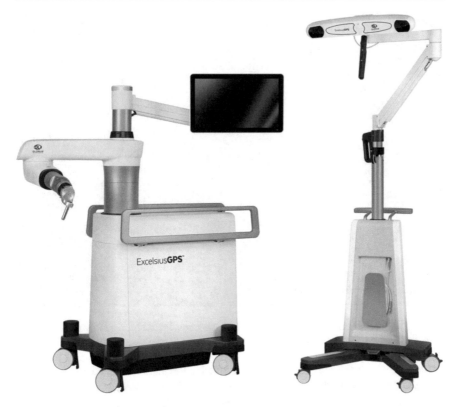

Fig. 2 The Excelsius GPS® (Globus Medical, Inc., Audubon, Pennsylvania) robotic surgical system. Image used with permission from Globus Medical, Inc.

2.4 Globus Medical: Excelsius GPS

The Excelsius GPS® (Globus Medical, Inc., Audubon, Pennsylvania), introduced in 2017, while similar to the ROSA and Mazor models, incorporates several design modifications to address errors introduced by movement (Fig. 2) [4]. The GPS automatically compensates for patient movement, and feedback is provided if the drill slides or the reference frame moves [4, 18]. Furthermore, it features direct screw insertion via an external arm, rendering K-wires unnecessary (Fig. 3). Because the GPS has been introduced very recently, it has been much less extensively studied than the SpineAssist.

2.5 Intuitive Surgical: da Vinci Surgical System

The da Vinci Surgical System® (Intuitive Surgical, Sunnyvale, California) was approved by the FDA in 2000 for laparoscopic procedures [1]. Unlike the shared-control model of the previously-mentioned robots, the da Vinci is a telesurgical

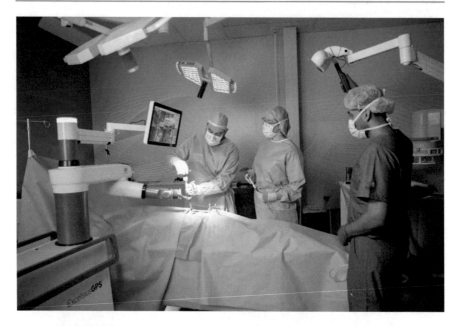

Fig. 3 The Excelsius GPS® (Globus Medical, Inc., Audubon, Pennsylvania) in the clinical setting. Image used with permission from Globus Medical, Inc.

system in which the surgeon operates remotely. Because it is used for a range of procedures outside of spine surgery, it has been widely studied, and it provides better visualization than conventional laparoscopy [4]. Benefits include tremor filtering, high definition video for the surgeon and staff, and multiple operating arms with a separate remote booth, ideal for trainees (Fig. 4) [1].

Primary reported uses for the da Vinci system in spine surgery include anterior lumbar interbody fusions (ALIF), resection of spinal tumors, and transoral odontoidectomies [4, 19, 20]. Early studies of laproscopic ALIF failed to demonstrate any benefit in clinical outcomes for patients such as blood loss, complications, and length of stay. This partly explains the relatively rare use of this procedure [4].

Even though the da Vinci robot has numerous advantages, areas for improvement remain, mostly related to the lack of diversity in instrument compatibility. The most pertinent of these disadvantages is the lack of instruments such as burrs and rongeurs to assist with bone dissection [21]. Thus, the da Vinci is not a viable tool for metastatic tumors with osseous involvement or primary bone tumors; it is better suited to soft tissue masses [21].

3   Accuracy of Implant Placement

Numerous recent studies have shown that robotic-assisted screw placement in spine surgery results in greater accuracy than conventional, free-hand placement [8, 22–25]. Kim et al. in 2017 published a randomized controlled trial comparing 37 patients receiving a robot-assisted posterior lumbar interbody fusion (PLIF) to 41

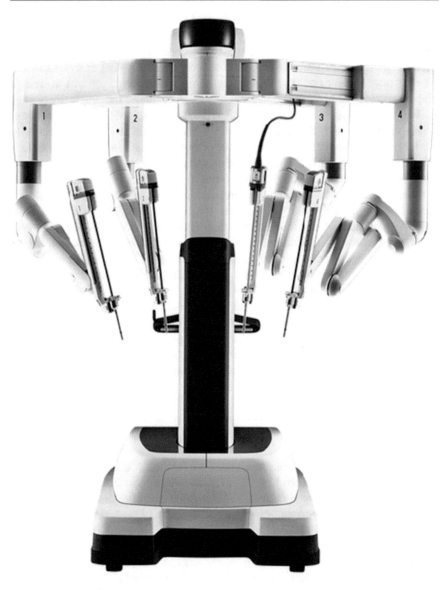

Fig. 4 The da Vinci Surgical System® (Intuitive Surgical, Sunnyvale, California). Image taken from https://commons.wikimedia.org/wiki/File:Davinci-xi-surgical-system.png, shared without changes under Creative Commons Attribution-Share Alike 3.0 Unported license. Accessed November 22, 2020

receiving free-hand PLIF, with primary endpoints of intrapedicular screw placement accuracy and proximal facet joint accuracy [22]. They found that the use of robotic assistance had no significant effect on intrapedicular accuracy but was associated with a decrease in violation of the proximal facet joint ($p < 0.001$). The authors noted that the free-hand technique for screw placement relies upon the surgeon's ability to coordinate the trajectory of the screw insertion in three planes solely on the basis of CT/fluoroscopy-based navigation, while the robotic system mechanically guides the surgeon to the exact planned trajectory independent of his/ her proficiency. A 2019 meta-analysis of randomized controlled trials by Li et al. demonstrated similar findings: use of the robot-assisted technique was associated with more accurate pedicle screw placement when evaluated radiologically [26].

To date, only one randomized controlled trial has shown a decreased accuracy of screw placement using the SpineAssist robot [7]. Ringel et al. implanted 298 pedicle screws in 60 patients requiring mono- or bi-segmental lumbar or lumbosacral stabilizations using a 1:1 ratio of conventional to robot-assisted placements. Ninety-three percent of conventionally placed screws had adequate accuracy (defined as cortical breach <2 mm in distance) compared to just 85% of screws placed with robotic assistance; this difference reached statistical significance ($p = 0.019$). The authors suggested several mechanisms that could explain why their results conflicted with most of the literature: (1) choice of robot fixation to the patient (securing a platform to a cranial spinous process with a single K-wire), which could have led to movement of the robot relative to the patient; (2) lateral skidding of the cannula for screw entry along the lateral aspect of the facet joint; or (3) other dislocations of the cannula, such as by local muscle tissue through which the cannula perforates. These mechanisms were considered by Kim et al., who attempted to minimize lateral skidding of the entry cannula by preparing the pedicle screw by the Peterson technique and opting for a lateral-to-medial screw trajectory [22]. Importantly, these screw malpositions, regardless of potential cause, were not associated with increased rates of revision surgeries.

4 Clinical Outcomes

Several prospective trials have examined the relationship between operative time and use of robotic assistance [14, 22, 27, 28]. While most individual trials have failed to demonstrate any significant difference in operative time between robot-assisted and traditional procedures, a meta-analysis by Li et al. showed that robotic assistance was associated with a longer operative time. However, robotic assistance was also associated with the same postoperative stay, visual analog scale scores, and Oswestry disability index scores [26]. A meta-analysis by Yu et al. yielded similar findings with respect to increased operative time in the robot-assisted group [9] and failed to demonstrate any significant association between rates of complications and robot-assisted approaches.

Notably, Yu et al. found that 100% of complications in the robot-assisted group were related to infection, while 75% of those in the conventional group were related to pedicle screw placement, suggesting that infection rates could be attributable to the increased operative time associated with robotic assistance [9]. Even in increasingly complex spinal surgeries, the available literature suggests that differences in complication rates are negligible. A retrospective comparison of conventional fluoroscopic-guided versus SpineAssist-treated patients undergoing surgery for thoracolumbar metastatic tumors revealed no differences in accuracy or postoperative infection rates [29].

While the literature is scant, small studies suggest several niche applications for robotic assistance in spine surgery such as sacroiliac (SI) screw placement, biopsies, vertebroplasties, and even S2 alar-iliac screw placement [30–33]. Owing to the complex anatomy of the pelvis, screw malposition rates in this region can reach as high as 15% [25]. One randomized controlled trial showed that robot-assisted procedures were associated with higher rates of screw accuracy than free-hand placement. Furthermore, in the robot-assisted procedures, the time for guidewire insertion was shorter than with free-hand placement; although there was no difference in overall operative time [25], probably owing to the increased preparation time for use of the robot. The increased range of freedom and capacity to pre-plan a procedure enables surgical robots to intervene in areas that are otherwise difficult to reach using a traditional, free-hand technique; Dreval et al. demonstrated the use of robotic assistance in vertebroplasties for fractures and hemangiomas with high accuracy and safety [11]. It has also been shown that robotic assistance decreases the incidence of intraoperative injury to the proximal facet joint, suggesting that it could help to minimize the risk for adjacent segment disease [34].

5 Radiation Exposure

The use of fluoroscopic visualization is common in spinal procedures for navigation to the surgical site and for assessing hardware position intraoperatively. Accordingly, spinal procedures can expose operating room staff on average to 10–12 times as much radiation as non-spinal procedures [35]. Over a career, a spine surgeon can see 50 times the lifetime radiation dose of a hip surgeon; ionizing radiation has been linked to development of complications such as cataracts, leukemia, and other cancers [1]. Although surgeons can minimize radiation exposure through protective equipment such as lead gowns, thyroid shields, and protective gloves, robot assistance shows promise in reducing this significant concern further [1]. A recent meta-analysis examining two prospective randomized controlled trials that studied intraoperative radiation exposure revealed that robotic assistance is associated with decreased overall intraoperative radiation exposure time and overall intraoperative radiation dose [24, 26, 28]. The protective effect of robotic assistance on radiation exposure is attributable to the preoperative and intraoperative trajectory planning that obviates the need for repeated fluoroscopy outside the initial preoperative preparation (Fig. 5).

6 Cost–Benefit Analysis

Some authors have proposed that the use of robotics in spine surgery can potentially result in cost savings because of decreased operative time, length of stay, exposure to ionizing radiation, and revision surgeries [12]. As discussed previously, a few meta-analyses have demonstrated associations between increased operative time and use of robotic assistance. However, some of these findings of increased

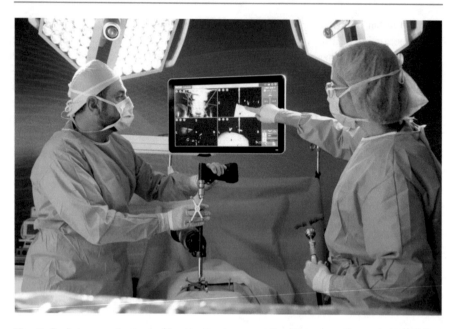

Fig. 5 Real-time navigation with the Excelsius GPS® (Globus Medical, Inc., Audubon, Pennsylvania) in the clinical setting, providing surgical site visualization without the need for excess radiation exposure. Image used with permission from Globus Medical, Inc.

operative time could be related to inexperience with robotics for spine procedures. Whether this effect will persist as the learning curves for use of the technology are traversed is yet to be determined. For example, despite meta-analyses of prospective randomized trials demonstrating increased operative times, a large retrospective study by Menger et al. concluded that patients receiving robot-assisted surgery had shorter length of stay, fewer revision surgeries, lower infection rates, and shorter operative time [36]. A prospective, multi-center trial is currently underway to identify any differences in surgical complication rates, rates of revisions, and radiation exposure using robotic assistance for various degenerative spine diseases; preliminary results indicate that robotic treatment is associated with fewer complications and revisions, although the follow-up period is not complete and the sample size is small [37]. Given the large costs for initial purchase and annual maintenance service on surgical robotics, popularization of robotic surgery in the future is likely to depend on robustly demonstrated efficacy in surgical outcomes such as minimization of revision operations, infections, and patient length of stay.

7   Conclusion

Robotic assistance in spine surgery, emerging recently as an adjunct for pedicle screw placement, has been shown in several clinical studies to confer higher accuracy, and also lower radiation exposure to the surgeon, than conventional techniques, without significantly affecting the complication rates. Although these initial results are promising, widespread adoption of robotics for spinal applications must first overcome fiscal barriers, as few available studies support cost-efficacy. Further clinical studies are needed to establish clear indications, limitations, and other areas of improvement for surgical robots in the spine subspecialty. Nevertheless, current robotic systems and further technological advancements show promise for expanding indications in spine surgery, especially for complex cases where increased dexterity and reproducibility are desirable to augment current surgical technique.

References

1. Overley SC, Cho SK, Mehta AI, Arnold PM. Navigation and robotics in spinal surgery: where are we now? Neurosurgery. 2017;80(3S):S86–99.
2. Sukovich W, Brink-Danan S, Hardenbrook M. Miniature robotic guidance for pedicle screw placement in posterior spinal fusion: early clinical experience with the SpineAssist. Int J Med Robot. 2006;2(2):114–22.
3. Chenin L, Peltier J, Lefranc M. Minimally invasive transforaminal lumbar interbody fusion with the ROSA(TM) spine robot and intraoperative flat-panel CT guidance. Acta Neurochir. 2016;158(6):1125–8.
4. D'Souza M, Gendreau J, Feng A, Kim LH, Ho AL, Veeravagu A. Robotic-assisted spine surgery: history, efficacy, cost. And Fut Trends Robot Surg. 2019;6:9–23.
5. Nooh A, Aoude A, Fortin M, Aldebeyan S, Abduljabbar FH, Eng PJ, et al. Use of computer assistance in lumbar fusion surgery: analysis of 15 222 patients in the ACS-NSQIP database. Global Spine J. 2017;7(7):617–23.
6. Devito DP, Kaplan L, Dietl R, Pfeiffer M, Horne D, Silberstein B, et al. Clinical acceptance and accuracy assessment of spinal implants guided with SpineAssist surgical robot: retrospective study. Spine (Phila Pa 1976). 2010;35(24):2109–15.
7. Ringel F, Stüer C, Reinke A, Preuss A, Behr M, Auer F, et al. Accuracy of robot-assisted placement of lumbar and sacral pedicle screws: a prospective randomized comparison to conventional freehand screw implantation. Spine (Phila Pa 1976). 2012;37(8):E496–501.
8. Le X, Tian W, Shi Z, Han X, Liu Y, Liu B, et al. Robot-assisted versus fluoroscopy-assisted cortical bone trajectory screw instrumentation in lumbar spinal surgery: a matched-cohort comparison. World Neurosurg. 2018;120:e745–e51.
9. Yu L, Chen X, Margalit A, Peng H, Qiu G, Qian W. Robot-assisted vs freehand pedicle screw fixation in spine surgery - a systematic review and a meta-analysis of comparative studies. Int J Med Robot. 2018;14(3):e1892.
10. Hu X, Lieberman IH. What is the learning curve for robotic-assisted pedicle screw placement in spine surgery? Clin Orthop Relat Res. 2014;472(6):1839–44.
11. Dreval' ON, Rynkov IP, Kasparova KA, Bruskin A, Aleksandrovskiĭ V, Zil'bernshteĭn V. Results of using spine assist Mazor in surgical treatment of spine disorders. ZhVoprNeirokhirIm N NBurdenko. 2014;78(3):14–20.
12. Fiani B, Quadri SA, Farooqui M, Cathel A, Berman B, Noel J, et al. Impact of robot-assisted spine surgery on health care quality and neurosurgical economics: a systemic review. Neurosurg Rev. 2020;43(1):17–25.
13. Hu X, Ohnmeiss DD, Lieberman IH. Robotic-assisted pedicle screw placement: lessons learned from the first 102 patients. Eur Spine J. 2013;22(3):661–6.
14. Kim HJ, Lee SH, Chang BS, Lee CK, Lim TO, Hoo LP, et al. Monitoring the quality of robot-assisted pedicle screw fixation in the lumbar spine by using a cumulative summation test. Spine (Phila Pa 1976). 2015;40(2):87–94.
15. Khan A, Meyers JE, Siasios I, Pollina J. Next-generation robotic spine surgery: first report on feasibility, safety, and learning curve. Oper Neurosurg (Hagerstown). 2019;17(1):61–9.
16. Suliman A, Wollstein R, Bernfeld B, Bruskin A. Robotic-assisted device in posterior spinal fusion for a high risk thoracolumbar fracture in ankylosing spondylitis. Asian Spine J. 2014;8(1):64–8.

17. Lefranc M, Peltier J. Evaluation of the ROSA™ spine robot for minimally invasive surgical procedures. Expert Rev Med Devices. 2016;13(10):899–906.
18. Zygourakis CC, Ahmed AK, Kalb S, Zhu AM, Bydon A, Crawford NR, et al. Technique: open lumbar decompression and fusion with the Excelsius GPS robot. Neurosurg Focus. 2018;45(Video Suppl 1):V6.
19. Lee JY, Bhowmick DA, Eun DD, Welch WC. Minimally invasive, robot-assisted, anterior lumbar interbody fusion: a technical note. J Neurol Surg A Cent Eur Neurosurg. 2013;74(4):258–61.
20. Bertelsen A, Melo J, Sánchez E, Borro D. A review of surgical robots for spinal interventions. Int J Med Robot. 2013;9(4):407–22.
21. Trybula SJ, Oyon DE, Wolinsky JP. Robotic tissue manipulation and resection in spine surgery. Neurosurg Clin N Am. 2020;31(1):121–9.
22. Kim HJ, Jung WI, Chang BS, Lee CK, Kang KT, Yeom JS. A prospective, randomized, controlled trial of robot-assisted vs freehand pedicle screw fixation in spine surgery. Int J Med Robot. 2017;13(3)
23. Lonjon N, Chan-Seng E, Costalat V, Bonnafoux B, Vassal M, Boetto J. Robot-assisted spine surgery: feasibility study through a prospective case-matched analysis. Eur Spine J. 2016;25(3):947–55.
24. Roser F, Tatagiba M, Maier G. Spinal robotics: current applications and future perspectives. Neurosurgery. 2013;72(Suppl 1):12–8.
25. Wang JQ, Wang Y, Feng Y, Han W, Su YG, Liu WY, et al. Percutaneous sacroiliac screw placement: a prospective randomized comparison of robot-assisted navigation procedures with a conventional technique. Chin Med J. 2017;130(21):2527–34.
26. Li HM, Zhang RJ, Shen CL. Accuracy of pedicle screw placement and clinical outcomes of robot-assisted technique versus conventional freehand technique in spine surgery from nine randomized controlled trials: a meta-analysis. Spine (Phila Pa 1976). 2020;45(2):E111–E9.
27. Han X, Tian W, Liu Y, Liu B, He D, Sun Y, et al. Safety and accuracy of robot-assisted versus fluoroscopy-assisted pedicle screw insertion in thoracolumbar spinal surgery: a prospective randomized controlled trial. J Neurosurg Spine. 2019;1-8
28. Hyun SJ, Kim KJ, Jahng TA, Kim HJ. Minimally invasive robotic versus open fluoroscopic-guided spinal instrumented fusions: a randomized controlled trial. Spine (Phila Pa 1976). 2017;42(6):353–8.
29. Solomiichuk V, Fleischhammer J, Molliqaj G, Warda J, Alaid A, von Eckardstein K, et al. Robotic versus fluoroscopy-guided pedicle screw insertion for metastatic spinal disease: a matched-cohort comparison. Neurosurg Focus. 2017;42(5):E13.
30. Bederman SS, Hahn P, Colin V, Kiester PD, Bhatia NN. Robotic GUIDANCE for S2-alar-iliac screws in spinal deformity correction. Clin Spine Surg. 2017;30(1):E49–53.
31. Hu X, Lieberman IH. Robotic-guided sacro-pelvic fixation using S2 alar-iliac screws: feasibility and accuracy. Eur Spine J. 2017;26(3):720–5.
32. Hyun SJ, Kim KJ, Jahng TA. S2 alar iliac screw placement under robotic guidance for adult spinal deformity patients: technical note. Eur Spine J. 2017;26(8):2198–203.
33. Laratta JL, Shillingford JN, Lombardi JM, Alrabaa RG, Benkli B, Fischer C, et al. Accuracy of S2 alar-iliac screw placement under robotic guidance. Spine Deform. 2018;6(2):130–6.
34. Kim HJ, Kang KT, Park SC, Kwon OH, Son J, Chang BS, et al. Biomechanical advantages of robot-assisted pedicle screw fixation in posterior lumbar interbody fusion compared with freehand technique in a prospective randomized controlled trial-perspective for patient-specific finite element analysis. Spine J. 2017;17(5):671–80.
35. Ravi B, Zahrai A, Rampersaud R. Clinical accuracy of computer-assisted two-dimensional fluoroscopy for the percutaneous placement of lumbosacral pedicle screws. Spine (Phila Pa 1976). 2011;36(1):84–91.
36. Menger RP, Savardekar AR, Farokhi F, Sin A. A cost-effectiveness analysis of the integration of robotic spine technology in spine surgery. Neurospine. 2018;15(3):216–24.
37. Schroerlucke S, Good C, Wang MA. Prospective, comparative study of robotic-guidance versus freehand in minimally invasive spinal fusion surgery: first report from MIS ReFRESH. Spine J. 2016;16(10)

Nanorobots in Neurosurgery

Lucas Capo and Jesus Lafuente

1 Introduction

Since the late twentieth century, neurosurgery has undergone a revolution in diagnosis and treatment owing to an explosion in technology. Technological developments in imaging guidance, intraoperative imaging, and microscopy have pushed neurosurgeons to the limits of their dexterity. The introduction of robotic-assisted surgery has provided surgeons with improved ergonomics and enhanced visualization, dexterity, and haptic capabilities.

Nanotechnology is defined as technology at the nanometer scale that can be used in the real world. The National Nanotechnology Initiative (NNI) defines this scale as encompassing elements between 1 and 100 nm. The relevance of this can be seen when it is recalled that a cell surface receptor measures approximately 40 nm, a DNA strand 2 nm and an albumin molecule around 7 nm [1].

Research in this innovative field will provide not only advances and discoveries of new materials but also possible advances in other fields such as medicine and health in general. Examples of the materials deployed in nanotechnologies include autoasambled molecular agglomerates using agents in solution, biological molecules such as DNA, etc.

Nanorobotics is the field of nanotechnology concerned with the design and creation of versatile robots at the molecular or cellular level. Such robots will allow us to access all the human body, performing new procedures at the cellular level and providing diagnostics and treatment with previously unimagined precision.

L. Capo
Sagrat Cor University Hospital, Barcelona, Spain

J. Lafuente (✉)
UAB (Autonomous University of Barcelona), Barcelona, Spain

Spine Unit at Hospital del Mar, Barcelona, Spain

© The Author(s), under exclusive license to Springer Nature
Switzerland AG 2022
M. M. Al-Salihi et al. (eds.), *Introduction to Robotics in Minimally Invasive Neurosurgery*, https://doi.org/10.1007/978-3-030-90862-1_6

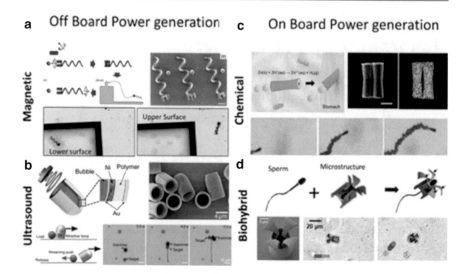

Fig. 1 Powering mechanism for micro/nanorobots. (**a**) Magnetically-propelled microrobot based on rotating microcoil. (**b**) Ultrasound-propelled microrobot powered by cavitating microbubble. (**c**) Chemically-propelled motor based on zinc microtube; the microrobot converts gastric fluid into gas bubbles that generate the propulsion thrust. (**d**) Biohybrid microrobot based on the integration of a sperm cell with a synthetic structure. Figure from: Soto F, Wang J, Ahmed R, Demirci U. Medical robotics: Medical micro/nanorobots in precision medicine (adv. Sci. 21/2020). Adv Sci (Weinh). 2020;7(21):2070117. (Obtained from "Open Access" sources under CC-BY license)

Movement of these nanorobots is the first challenge; traditional battery components are not possible at such a small scale. Options currently being considered are: chemically powered engines, magnetic swimmers, electrical, thermal and optical energy, or combinations of those to produce hybrid nanorobots. These principles of nanorobotic motion have led to the development of different nanorobots such as micro-rockets, helicoidal swimmers, ultrasound impulse nanocables, and even hybrid microrobots driven by sperm cells (Fig. 1).

Recent studies have demonstrated the potential use of these prototypes in such areas as target delivery, precision surgery, sensing biological agents, and detoxification.

This chapter will discuss the use of these nanorobots in a high-precision surgical field such as neuroscience, including neurosurgery.

2 Nanorobots for Precision Surgery

The use of robotic technology to assist surgeons was described conceptually almost 30 years ago but has only recently become feasible. The intrinsic characteristics of robots such as high precision, repeatability, and endurance make them the ideal surgeon assistants and have led surgeons to develop less invasive and more precise techniques. However, the challenge remains of producing robots that can be introduced into the body, reaching areas that have hitherto been impossible to reach. It will open a new paradigm for the development of novel diagnosis and treatment techniques [2].

Untethered tools such as nano-drills, micro-forceps, and micro-bullets are some of the elements that could face limitations in microscopic surgery.

Nanorobots directed by different forms of energy are capable of obtaining cellular tissue biopsies and of navigating the entire human body, since they can pass through vascular capillaries and work at a cellular level. Untethered micro-forceps represent a huge leap in the autonomy of these nanorobots; they can grasp and remove tissue in a similar way to the forceps that we use routinely. They can also respond automatically to grasping the tissue by changing shape in response to micro-ambience changes such as pH differences, temperature changes, or the activities of local enzymes. However, such changes will not interfere with the preservation of the tissue obtained, allowing it to be recovered and examined properly (Fig. 2).

Magnetically impulsed nanorobots have also been proposed since magnetic impulses can pass through thicker tissues. A clear example is magnetic rotational microdrills, which have shown a high index of penetration in such tissues. At the same time, the magnetic fields created are used to navigate the nanorobot. Figure 3 shows several examples including nanobots injected into the vitreous cavity through a surgical opening in the eye. A magnetic bovine system was used to allow the nanorobot to navigate to the posterior segment of a rabbit eye.

As well as magnetic fields, ultrasound has been proposed for the development of micro-bullets. These consist of biocompatible fuel and are greatly accelerated by ultrasound, allowing them to penetrate, ablate, and destroy tissues [3].

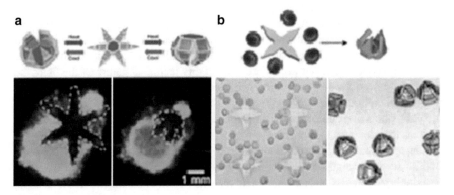

Fig. 2 Microrobot-based biopsy and sampling. (**a**) Star-shaped gripper collecting tissue. (**b**) Star gripper collecting red blood cells. Figure from: Soto F, Wang J, Ahmed R, Demirci U. Medical robotics: Medical micro/nanorobots in precision medicine (adv. Sci. 21/2020). Adv Sci (Weinh). 2020;7(21):2070117. (Obtained from "Open Access" sources under CC-BY license)

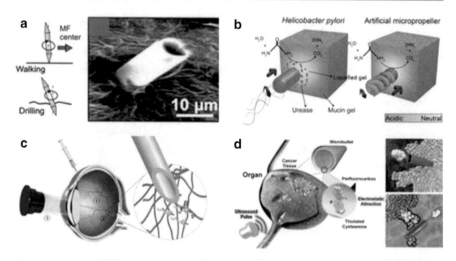

Fig. 3 Micro/nanorobots for tissue penetration. (**a**) Magnetic microdrill entering liver tissue. (**b**) Magnetic microdrill penetrating mucin gel. (**c**) Magnetic microdrill mobilizing inside the eye. (**d**) Ultrasound powered microbullet for tissue penetration and cleaving. Figure from: Soto F, Wang J, Ahmed R, Demirci U. Medical robotics: Medical micro/nanorobots in precision medicine (adv. Sci. 21/2020). Adv Sci (Weinh). 2020;7(21):2070117. (Obtained from "Open Access" sources under CC-BY license)

3   Neuroscience Applications

Although robotics has provided invaluable assistance in other surgical specialties, access and the very delicate nature of neurological tissue have remained obstacles against using this technology in the brain.

However, neurological surgery is well suited for incorporating robotic assistance. Traditionally, several aspects of our subspecialty lend themselves to the need for and implementation of robotics, including: the rich history of neurosurgical innovation in stereotaxy and navigated localization; the established anatomical confines that are protected by and oriented very specifically toward bony structures; the microsurgical nature of our procedures; the highly technical nature of the field; the growth and need for growth in minimally invasive neurosurgery; and a culture that adopts and embraces new technology.

Nanorobots overcome most of the limitations mentioned above, providing access to areas that not even the human eye can reach.

The application of nanorobots to the human brain has been named "neural nanorobotics." Its medical applications will depend on its ability to monitor electric activity and single neuron synaptic activity in real time, as well as collecting information about neurotransmitter traffic and other data without injuring any surrounding tissue.

If a nanorobot with cellular repair capacity could be created, it would be able to treat most if not all pathologies of the central nervous system, particularly focusing on degenerative diseases such as Parkinson, Alzheimer, etc. [4, 5]. Furthermore, application of this technology should be useful not only for diagnosing and treating diseases but also for increasing the cognitive capacities of the human brain significantly. It is likely that during the next 30 years we will be able to develop nanorobots safe enough for real-time interface tasks between the human brain and biological (another brain) and non-biological computing systems, thus creating brain-to-brain interfaces (BTBI) and brain–computer interfaces (BCI), in particular brain–cloud interfaces (B/CI).

BTBI and BCI technologies could yield treatment for paralyzed patients, while B/CI will allow us access to the omnipresent pool of information (networks, servers, and databases). This will enable communications between persons and computers to be changed radically, thus producing a true cognitive empowerment of humanity. To develop these interfaces, three different types of neuro nanorobots have been proposed, each acting at a different level and at the same time with an external computer system. These are called Endoneurorobots, Gliabots, and Synaptobots. They are 0.5–10 nm in size and are introduced into the human body transdermally. They will travel toward and cross the blood–brain barrier to enter the CNS. Endoneurobots will enter the neural soma while Gliobots will enter the glial cells, and Synaptobots will remain between the axonal terminals, monitoring the synaptic gap and the neurotransmitters.

4   Brain–Machine Interface Applications

The brain–machine interface is a collaboration between a brain and a device that enables signals from that brain to direct and control some external activity such a cursor or a prosthetic limb. It enables a direct communication pathway between the brain and the object to be controlled.

The term "brain–machine interface" was coined in 1973 by Jacques J Vidal, a Belgian researcher working at UCLA. However, Professor Jonathan Wolpaw developed a brain–computer interface using electrodes in the surface of the skull instead of directly in the brain. The year 1998 marked a significant development in the field of brain mapping when Phillip Kennedy implanted the first brain–computer interface object into a human.

The development of a brain–computer interface allows us to restore previously lost functions in patients. Neuronal implants collect information from nerve cells that are then interpreted by an external computer, allowing a command to be executed to either a prosthesis or a computer. This mechanism allows people with limb paralysis to control their robotic prosthesis or people with "locked-in syndrome" to communicate through a computer screen, writing, sending messages, etc. (Fig. 4).

Nanorobots also allows us to perform surgical procedures at an axonal level. This could potentially restore lost neurological functions in a nerve plexus or at a spinal cord level following trauma. These robots can manipulate axons through electrophoresis, approach the damaged ends, or even glue them together through electrofusion, opening a door into a new dimension of neurosurgical precision at a neural or axonal level [6].

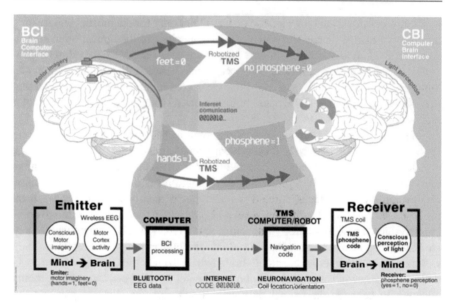

Fig. 4 Brain-to-brain interface (BTBI) for information transfer between human subjects. The emitter subject is shown on the left, where sensorimotor cortex activity was recorded using EEG electrodes. The emitter performed an imagery-based binary motor task: imagery of the feet (bit value 0) versus imagery of the hands (bit value 1). The receiver subject is shown on the right. The TMS coil was positioned differently over the visual cortex for 1 and 0 bit values, respectively, evoking or not evoking phosphenes (flashes of light). An Internet link was used for this brain-to-brain communication. Figure from: Martins NRB, Angelica A, Chakravarthy K, et al. Human brain/cloud interface. Front Neurosci. 2019;13:112. (Obtained from "Open Access" sources under CC-BY license)

5   Brain–Cloud Applications

Connecting your brain to a cloud seems far-fetched, but professors at the University of Berkley and the US Institute of Molecular Manufacturing suggest that this idea is not necessarily implausible. Researchers predict that advances in nanotechnology, nanomedicine, artificial intelligence (AI), and computation could lead to a system in which areas of the human brain (neurons and synapses) are connected to cloud computing networks in real time. Furthermore, designed neural nanorobots could transmit data wirelessly to and from a cloud-connected supercomputer.

The supposed benefits of a human brain–cloud interface (B/CI) include improvement in education and in collective human intelligence.

In our current world, it is impossible to keep up with the exponential growth of available information and its associated learning and training; humans have biological limitations. Neural nanorobots will enable us to overcome these limitations, allowing our learning capacities to expand exponentially. However, the transmission of information and knowledge will not resolve everything, as knowledge requires analysis and interpretation; an increase in learning capacity does not necessarily entail an increase in creativity and imagination.

Research has demonstrated that people with higher IQs have more complex, more integrated, and more distant neural connections within and among brain regions than people with lower IQs. In these cases, a nanorobot-mediated B/CI could substantially increase intelligence, pattern recognition, and memory creating complex biological and non-biological networks.

The creation of virtual reality indistinguishable from reality itself has been advocated as a potential future application of nanorobot-mediated B/VI; furthermore, another person's life could be experienced through their eyes using connections in the same networks. However, these future prospects raise many ethical questions [7].

6 Clinical Trials in Neuro Oncology

Although most of the technical aspects of nanorobotics have been developed in animals, we wish to share our experience of one of the first human-based studies, currently under review by the European Agency pending a European grant. The study is: Innovative nanomaterials targeting bone metastases of the spine by two hits: inhibition of tumor progression and bone regeneration (INNATA). The aim of this study is to develop innovative treatments for inhibiting the progression of spinal metastases and simultaneously leading to the formation of new, healthy, and mechanically competent bone tissue. The main goal of the dual-functional anticancer and osteoinductive injectable nanostructure will be achieved through the following specific objectives: (1) synthesis of biocompatible hydrogels; (2) penetration by polymer nanosheets (NS) loaded with anticancer compounds (GO; ILs); (3) development of therapeutic injectable NS; (4) in vitro study to evaluate the anticancer, osteoinductive and angiogenic properties of NS; (5) in vivo validation to assess the anticancer and bone regenerative efficacies of the injectable therapeutic NS.

7 Limitations

There is a huge amount of research in this new technology. Despite the numerous efforts and capital investment, currently available resources impose limitations. One of the main limitations for applying these technologies is the safety and biocompatibility of nanorobots. Ideally, they should access the human body through intradermal injection, enter the vascular circulation, achieve the task for which they are designed, and then degrade either through the microbiological micro-ambiance or by excretion. Another very important aspect is the choice of materials for nanorobot design, since changes in their surfaces could induce intrinsic inflammatory reactions, reducing their life expectancy, minimizing their efficacy or even eliciting unwanted immunological responses.

Current preclinical studies are analyzing these two aspects, biocompatibility and security, as well as adequate materials for nanorobot production. These preclinical studies involve animal testing, and we are on the verge of implementing them in humans.

The next step should be to provide the infrastructure for mass production for these nanorobotic systems, concurrently with the design of new biocompatible materials through developments in tissue and molecular engineering. Similarly, the creation of new methods for generating motion as well as magnetic auto-assembly, magnetic levitation, etc. will make nanorobots more versatile and secure, eventually hiding them from the immune system of the patient [8].

8　Ethical Considerations

Individual personality and character is determined partly by genetics and partly by training and life experiences, collected and stored in the brain. Although the new technology is designed to access highly eloquent regions within the brain with few or no complications, the fact that it can potentially interfere with individual and personal characteristics raises huge ethical issues, which surely will have to be considered by the numerous regulatory agencies such as FDA, EMA, etc.

It is for this reason, as well as the high cost of such technology, that nanorobotics remains a promising field at a very early stage.

However, the specialty of neurological surgery is likely to overcome many major milestones in robotic technology over the coming years. Our history has already been intricately intertwined with the predecessors of today's nascent robotic platforms. This will make our future much like our past, one that is rich in scientific and technological advances.

9　Conclusion

It is likely that in the non-distant future we will be able to develop nanorobots safe enough for real-time interface tasks between the human brain and biological and non-biological computing systems, thus creating brain-to-brain interfaces and brain-computer interfaces, in particular brain-cloud interfaces. Current preclinical studies are analyzing biocompatibility and security, as well as adequate materials for nanorobot production. It is a fact that this technology can potentially interfere with individual and personal characteristics raise huge ethical issues, which surely will have to be considered by numerous regulatory agencies. It is for this reason, as well as the high cost of such technology, that nanorobotics remains a promising field at a very early stage.

References

1. Saadeh Y, Vyas D. Nanorobotic applications in medicine: current proposals and designs. Am J Robot Surg. 2014;1(1):4–11.
2. Bhushan B. Introduction to nanotechnology. In: Springer handbook of nanotechnology. Berlin Heidelberg: Springer; 2017. p. 1–19.
3. Sensing JL, Bertaesteban-Fernándezde Á, Wei G, Liangfang Z, Joseph W. Micro/nanorobots for biomedicine: delivery, surgery. Sci Robot. Published online. 2017.
4. Lafuente JV, Requejo C, Ugedo L. Nanodelivery of therapeutic agents in Parkinson's disease. Prog Brain Res. 2019;245:263–79.
5. Ozkizilcik A, Sharma A, Lafuente JV, et al. Nanodelivery of cerebrolysin reduces pathophysiology of Parkinson's disease. Prog Brain Res. 2019;245:201–46.
6. Chang WC, Hawkes EA, Kliot M, Sretavan DW. In vivo use of a nanoknife for axon microsurgery. Neurosurgery. 2007;61(4):683–91. discussion 691–2
7. Martins NRB, Angelica A, Chakravarthy K, et al. Human brain/cloud interface. Front Neurosci. 2019;13:112.
8. Soto F, Wang J, Ahmed R, Demirci U. Medical robotics: medical micro/nanorobots in precision medicine. Adv Sci (Weinh). 2020;7(21):2070117.

Artificial Intelligence and the Internet of Things in the Neurosurgical Operating Theater

Mohammed Maan Al-Salihi, Maryam Sabah Al-Jebur, and Tetsuya Goto

1 Introduction

Recently, with the onset of the fourth industrial revolution, represented by artificial intelligence (AI), big data, the Internet of Things (IoT), and robotics, interest in medical AI has increased more than ever [1, 2]. AI, the ability of a machine to think and learn, has undergone a revolution of applications from autonomous vehicles on our roads to digital personal assistants in our homes [3, 4]. It was introduced to medical disciplines via machine learning (ML), and neurosurgery has benefited most from AI-driven technological innovations, especially the subspecialty of functional and stereotactic neurosurgery [5]. Neurosurgical applications of AI that automate the diagnosis and treatment of movement-related disorders and epilepsy include: diagnostic brain imaging classification, preoperative planning, prediction of postoperative patient outcomes, location of epileptogenic zones within the brain, and selecting surgical candidates; in addition to automated surgical adjuncts, and autonomous surgical robots [6]. Such applications have the potential to enhance accuracy and save neurosurgeons' time [7]. Nevertheless, although AI and ML have been actively studied, few surgeons understand their basic concepts [8].

Similarly, few surgeons are familiar with IoT and digital biomarkers. IoT, composed of devices containing embedded sensors, is defined as any network of physical objects that contain embedded technology to communicate, sense, and interact with either their internal states or the external environment [9]. Although IoT and AI were previously defined separately, IoT has recently evolved as a technology including medical AI [10], and is widely used in medical fields [11–13]. Recent

M. M. Al-Salihi (✉) · M. S. Al-Jebur
College of Medicine, University of Baghdad, Baghdad, Iraq

T. Goto
Department of Neurosurgery, St. Marianna University School of Medicine, Kawasaki, Kanagawa, Japan
e-mail: tegotou@marianna-u.ac.jp

© The Author(s), under exclusive license to Springer Nature Switzerland AG 2022
M. M. Al-Salihi et al. (eds.), *Introduction to Robotics in Minimally Invasive Neurosurgery*, https://doi.org/10.1007/978-3-030-90862-1_7

studies in neurosurgery measuring physical activity in spinal patients have used various devices and sensors to monitor such patients in real time [14]. Such monitoring facilitates diagnosis and prompts treatment, which in turn lowers medical expenses [15]. The principle of IoT is that devices containing embedded sensors continually gather information from the environment and deliver it to a gateway via a wireless network, which receives this information from the sensors of the various devices and delivers it to a cloud that gathers, interprets, and stores that abundance of data in real time [16]. The OPeLiNK monitor is an intraoperatively applied communication interface through which the next-generation networked surgical operating room was built, known as the Smart Cyber Operating Theater (SCOT) (Figs. 1 and 2) [17]. The SCOT innovation offers the ability to interconnect the many devices in the neurosurgical operating room, integrating surgical information such as images of the surgical field, anesthetic data, visual evoked potential (*VEP*) monitoring, and navigation and biometric data, and displaying it all to a "Strategy Desk" in the operation room in the same timeline, which supports surgeons' decision making (Fig. 3) [17]. There is also control room beside the SCOT operating room that contains the MRI control desk and OPeLiNK server. The connection between the OPeLiNK server and other apparatus is an Ethernet cable built within the central wall to avoid interference with the intraoperative MRI (Figs. 4, 5, and 6).

This system has been highly mechanized and is used for both microscopic and endoscopic neurosurgery [17], proving extremely helpful in determining the appropriate extent of resection for malignant brain tumors and thus preserving neurological function (Fig. 7) [18].

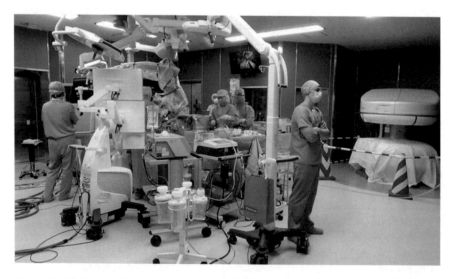

Fig. 1 The SCOT operation room; intraoperative MRI is installed in the same room. MRI, bipolar coagulator, a navigation system, and microscope are connected to the OPeLiNK through an Ethernet cable

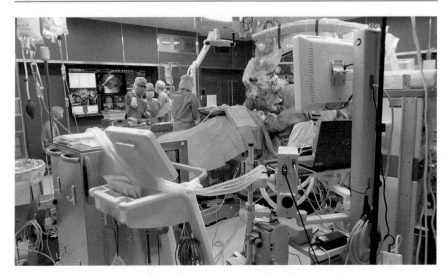

Fig. 2 The opposite side of the SCOT operation room. Anesthetic systems are also connected to the OPeLinK. The 60-inch 4K monitor at the wall displays all the information of the OPeLink. For the information on the monitor, "live" or "review" can be selected. The surgeon communicates with the strategy desk through this monitor

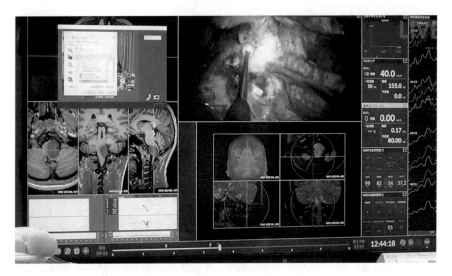

Fig. 3 The wall monitor of the OPeLinK; communication with the strategy desk, which appears on the left upper part of the picture. The navigation information appears on the left lower part of the picture, the microscopic view appears on the central upper part. The central lower part and the lowest line bar of the picture display the task history recording system. The task history can be placed not only the in the timeline bar but also in the navigation system. Infusion pump, anesthetic information, patient's general condition, and electrophysiological monitoring display (waveform of the ABR) all appear on the right side of the picture. This picture indicates the live mode. (It is difficult to judge whether this information is live or review)

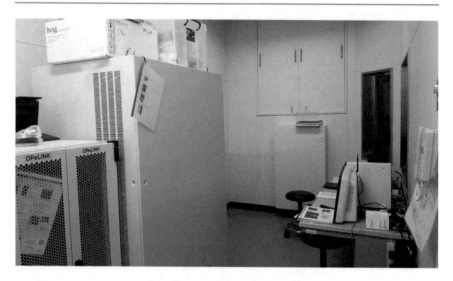

Fig. 4 Control room beside the SCOT operation room; MRI control desk on the right side, OPeLinK server on the left. The cable connecting the OPeLinK server and each item of apparatus is built within the central wall to avoid interference with the intraoperative MRI. The connecting system is not Wi-Fi; an Ethernet cable is used

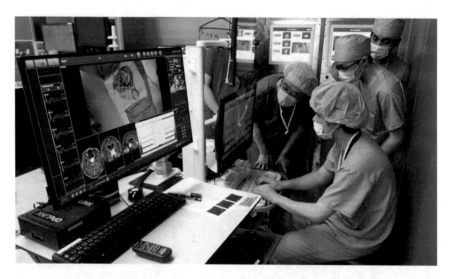

Fig. 5 Control desk of the wall monitor for OPeLinK on the left side of the picture, electrophysiological monitoring system on the right

In this chapter we will introduce the basic concepts of AI and IoT and their current and future-driven technological innovations in the neurosurgical field. We will also describe the basis on which the innovative new operating room, SCOT, was developed and applied in neurosurgery.

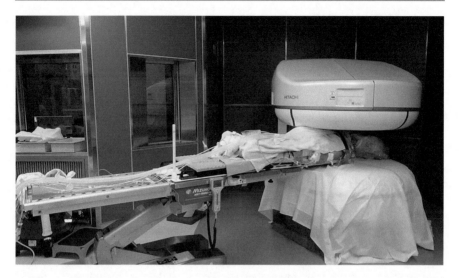

Fig. 6 Intraoperative MRI; no need to transfer the patient to another room. Data are updated to the navigation system directly

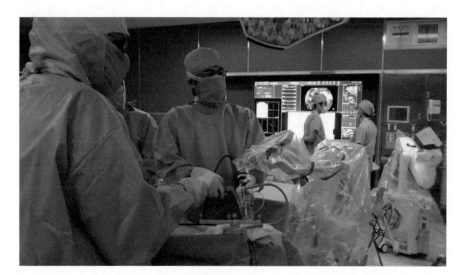

Fig. 7 Endoscopic neurosurgery operations are also performed in the SCOT operation room

2 Artificial Intelligence in Neurosurgery

2.1 Artificial Intelligence, Machine Learning, and Automation in Neurosurgery

Artificial intelligence (AI) is the branch of computer science that deals with the simulation of intelligent behavior by computers [19]. A significant subset of AI is machine learning (ML), the domain that allows computer algorithms to be trained and learn patterns by studying large amounts of data directly, without the need for rigid programming for each separate task (Table 1) [20]. Interestingly, in our daily lives, AI is already widely applied via ML and used inconspicuously in many applications including search and online shopping suggestions, speech recognition by smartphones, and email spam filters [4]. Likewise, AI and ML methods have entered medicine, have been tested in a variety of clinical applications, and have begun to establish capabilities approximating those of specialist physicians [21, 22], covering all phases of medical care and surgical fields: diagnosis, surgical planning, decision making, reducing intraoperative surgical workflow, prediction of patients' outcomes, efficiency enhancement, and postoperative reporting [3, 10, 23–28].

Table 1 Machine learning models of supervised, unsupervised, and reinforcement learning in clinical tasks

ML models	Algorithms	Mechanism	Applications
Supervised learning	• *Support vector machines (SVMs)* • *Random forests (RF)* • *Artificial neural networks (ANNs)* • Naive Bayesian	• Trained using known training dataset • Infer the predictions • Predict future outcomes	• Clinical prediction, such as treatment outcome • Prognostication
Unsupervised learning	• *K-means* • Fuzzy C-means • *Hierarchical clustering*	• Dataset is not classified or labeled • Tasked with identifying clustering values • Cannot make prediction • Model the underlying structure or distribution of the data qualitatively	• Diagnostics: Identify symptom clusters/ pattern identification of imaging data • Help in treatment strategies • Patient selection
Reinforcement learning	• Monte Carlo • Q-learning • State–action– reward–state– action (SARSA)	• Trained by reward and punishment • Determine the ideal behavior within a specific context based on simple reward on their actions	• Allocation tasks • Patients discharge selection • Algorithm control for surgical adjuncts and robotics

Data from Traverso, Alberto & Dankers, Frank & Osong, Biche & Wee, Leonard & Kuijk, Sander (2019). Diving Deeper into Models. https://doi.org/10.1007/978-3-319-99,713-1_9

Since developments in neurosurgery have always relied on cutting-edge technology, clinical implementations of AI have offered significant assistance especially for the subspecialties of spinal, vascular, and oncological surgery [10, 28, 29]. This is leading to AI-facilitated automation, a forthcoming technological revolution in medicine that is anticipated to lower costs, reduce medical errors, expand access to healthcare, and increase patient autonomy [30–32], not only in non-interventional aspects of medical care, but also potentially in the operating room and interventions, if it is applied along with surgical robotics [32] and operative adjuncts [33, 34].

Current diagnostic techniques produce large volumes of data that need investigation, extraction, and gross interpretation by trained specialists at high levels of sensitivity and specificity. Human interpretation is not always well suited to quantitative analysis of large noisy data volumes [30, 31], because it is impossible for a human to compare and analyze every voxel quantitatively in every slice from MRI or CT data. The application of ML-automated techniques using artificial neural networks to analyze radiological data can achieve faster and more accurate quantitative processing of these data at higher resolutions and speeds than is humanly possible [35–37]. Since ML uses every voxel as an individual input feature, the amount of data extracted is extremely high [20].

In addition, computer-aided data analysis can be one of the first ML applications for diagnosis, segmentation, or outcome prediction since its clinical application is noninvasive [3, 38]. One example of this potential ability is the prediction of molecular expression in gliomas using only MRI data; previously, invasive tissue sampling was required for molecular-level analysis [35, 39].

Therefore, the potential applications of AI in medicine and neuroscience are wide-ranging and are reinforced by the big data generated and stored in the modern clinical environment, where specific algorithms can be applied to analyze multimodal clinical data sources such as lab reports, alpha-numeric electronic health records, 2-dimensional and 3-dimensional radiological scans, and clinical images. According to the technique used, AI can automate and enhance implementation, administration, regulation, and clinical tasks, consequently reducing the human work burden, improving accuracy, and eliminating errors [40].

2.1.1 Non-interventional Applications

Non-interventional neurosurgical applications of AI automation for diagnosis include diagnostic brain imaging classification from sequence selection to image interpretation [41, 42], with rapid detection of certain conditions [24]. Several studies have reported the application of AI algorithms to imaging sequences to automate tumor classification [43], diagnose acute ischemic events [24] or aneurysms [29], and predict glioma features [35, 44]. In addition, automation has approximated the diagnostic performance of specialist physicians in neuropathology, particularly regarding genomic analysis [45] and tissue histopathology [46], electrophysiology [47], and analysis of electronic health records [40]. Also, recent retrospective studies have reported that these algorithms are superior to physicians at decision making tasks including preoperative planning and outcome prediction [48–50]. Regarding preoperative planning, several studies have compared ML with physicians [48,

51–55].Applications have included automated tumor segmentation [56], location of epileptogenic zones [43, 51–53], and selection of surgical candidates among pediatric epilepsy patients using ML-based natural language processing [54]. ML has also been used for calculating the vasospasm risk following subarachnoid hemorrhage [57], and predicting tissue injury and the effect of treatment for acute ischemic stroke [58]. ML models had a higher segmentation speed, with a median of 36–40 s rather than 20.2 min in manual segmentation [20]. In the four studies locating epileptogenic zones [43, 51–53], ML achieved significantly higher accuracy in differentiating between left-sided and right-sided temporal lobe epilepsy (TLE) based on functional MRI [53], whereas comparisons based on genetic information and symptoms failed to differentiate TLE from extra-temporal lobe epilepsy [43]. Automation also enhanced outcome prediction by predicting survival rates in neuro-oncology on the basis of MRI features [48, 49], and in traumatic brain injury on the basis of clinical features [57], thus helping in treatment selection and boosting patient stratification.

However, clinical use of ML models could displace clinicians, the so-called human vs. machine paradigm. In practice, even though ML models are enabled to perform a given analysis with much higher accuracy, clinicians must still be considered. A systematic review has reported that ML models were better when used to assist the clinician in decision making, which is then called "human-and-machine." [20] In four studies that assessed the combined performances of clinicians along with ML models for radiological diagnosis or segmentation, the results suggested that ML combined with clinician decision making was superior to ML models alone or clinician decision making alone [52, 59]. This demonstrates that ML models and human specialists complement each other [20].

A barrier to the application of ML models in practice is the large body of adequately categorized and complete data needed to generate such models. Thus, because higher quality data are used, the performance of ML models in research settings could be overestimated in relation to their true performance in their clinical setting. Another hurdle is the rightly restricted access to patients' data, referred to as privacy considerations, which make it difficult to obtain high volume training data sets [60]. To overcome these barriers, further studies should consider the human-and-machine approach in order to discover how the powerful analyses that ML offers can best enhance the work of clinicians. Also, efforts are needed to create a legal and ethical framework that supports the collection of training data, validation, and regulation of the performance of ML models before and after their deployment in clinical care [20].

2.1.2 Interventional Applications

ML can potentially help with interventions in neurosurgery through controlling the mechanisms of operative adjuncts and autonomous surgical robots, permitting the interventions to be more precise with minimal surgical errors. Neurosurgical adjuncts are designed to maximize both the accuracy and freedom of the intervention with least collateral damage. Therefore, since the adjunct's performance depends on the human using it, considering that the surgeon's unaided performance relies on various physical and mental factors, approximately 23.7% to 27.8% of neurosurgical mistakes result from the surgeon's poor technique [61]. For that reason, surgical adjuncts such as semi-automated operating microscopes and endoscopes, which are capable of automated self-positioning, are potentially useful in spinal and intracranial procedures [33, 34]; automated image guidance [62], which applies imaging data acquired preoperatively or intraoperatively, helps in planning techniques for the operative trajectory [63, 64]; and together with other potentially automated surgical adjuncts used to alert surgeons when they encroach upon critical structures [65], these will all maximize the rapidity and accuracy of interventions, minimizing the technical errors and collateral damage secondary to human factors, and thus minimizing postoperative deficits.

Moreover, interventional tasks could be partially or even fully automated in the near future, thanks to the possibility of combining robot-assisted devices with AI automated control algorithms, along with advanced sensory technology including machine vision, haptic and motion sensors, and kinematics. These have made it possible to automate soft-tissue interventional surgery [66–68], and can augment human surgical capability beyond its current limits. During the past 15 years, robotic systems have developed exponentially to provide greater degrees of freedom, better orientation and positioning of surgical instrumentation, and superior three-dimensional vision, in addition to their greatest contributions: eliminating trembling, improving resolution, reducing operative time, and imposing physical restrictions to avoid vulnerable areas [69]. However, they usually have to be controlled by humans in real time. Regular common robotic systems include PUMA 200, introduced in 1985, the first robot implemented in the neurosurgical operating room to perform a brain biopsy successfully [70]. Ever since then, applications of robotized systems have progressed to include ventricular catheter placement, radiosurgery, placement of electrodes in deep brain stimulation or of stereo-electroencephalographic electrodes for investigating refractory epilepsy, and laser ablation [71–74]. Many different systems have been prototyped and become either commercially available, under trial, or discontinued [75]. Already, currently active commercially available neurosurgical robots include Neuromate (Renishaw-Mayfield SA., Nyon, Switzerland), first developed in 1987 [76]; SurgiScope (ISIS Robotics, Saint Martin d'Heres, France), a delta parallel microscope-carrying robot, reported in 2003 [77]; ROSA (MedTech SA., Montpellier, France), the first to implant electrodes for deep brain stimulation [78]; and Renaissance (Mazor Robotics, Caesarea, Israel), a partly autonomous device that uses preoperative imaging to guide operative trajectories in placing pedicle screws [79]. However, the classification of such robots according to surgeon–robot interaction included only three models: (1) the supervisory controlled system, in which the robot autonomously follows a surgical plan made under the supervision of the doctor using CT or MRI scans of the patient brain; (2) the tele-operated system, in which the robot replicates the surgeon's movement in real time using a haptic system interface; (3) the shared control system, a symbiotic system in which the surgeon has complete control while the robot acts only as an assistant, the surgeon's hand using the instrument to prevent tremors and ensure safety in delicate surgical areas [80]. Although neurosurgical robots can potentially save surgeons time and simplify complex procedures, the recent conjoining of AI control algorithms with the evident capabilities of surgical robots can create a fourth fully automated model of surgical robotics that could further enhance surgical capability, improve outcomes, and increase potential care access without human intervention [68]. Shademan et al. reported a complete porcine intestinal anastomosis performed in vivo by an autonomous surgical robot, the Smart Tissue Autonomous Robot (STAR) [68, 81]. Future autonomous robots could potentially observe, think, and act independently of active human intervention. However, surgical robots can be automated through teaching via ML, either explicitly by direct programming, implicitly by the robot watching a surgeon or a video or by training it in virtual reality [32]. Although effectively outperforming the human expert, the robot must also be able to evaluate all relevant sensory inputs such as the tactile and visual features of the surgical field and the positional information, and must be able to access a database detailing how to achieve the surgical goal safely. Accordingly, a combination of implicit and the explicit techniques will be necessary, with continual modifications and reinforcement by surgeons [82]. The tasks for an autonomous surgical robot then range between the following three parameters: human independence, mission complexity, and environmental difficulty [83]. AI cannot yet be mediated to provide an autonomous system representing motion sequences or surgical videos simply, or to learn all arbitrarily complex multi-layered tasks. However, decomposition of those complex surgical tasks into simpler motions and subtasks could facilitate the analysis of human exemplars [84]. The da Vinci system, using motion and video recordings, has segmented robotic surgical motions [85]. In addition, deep learning techniques have been used for segmentation; non-surgical image libraries were used to teach the pre-trained architectures [86]. However, segmentation of surgical tasks remains an open problem owing to the difficulty of providing highly variable time-series data. For the further research needed to solve this, Intuitive Surgical Inc. and Johns Hopkins University have proposed a dataset for surgical activity consisting of available motion and video data [87]. Nevertheless, some autonomous robotic systems outside of neurosurgery have successfully accomplished isolated surgical tasks based on exemplary datasets provided by humans [88]. Also, the EndoPAR system, using a database of recurrent neural networks from 25 surgeons' trajectories, has accomplished knot-tying tasks autonomously [89]. Multilateral subtasks such as debridement and pattern cutting have also been automated using learning by observation [90]. Finally, the KUKA LWR platform has performed autonomous microanastomosis using learning based on demonstration of techniques [68]. Partially autonomous surgical robotics already in use are Mazor X, which calculates and guides operative trajectories using preoperative imaging for pedicle screw placement [79], and CyberKnife, the first system used for frameless stereotactic radiosurgery; it remains the only commercially available truly autonomous surgical robot that treats tumors [91]. Supervised autonomous robots could yet represent the most promising surgical model of autonomy, encompassing a symbiotic combination of man's interventional reinforcement and high-level supervision, and the machine's skill at performing precise motions [84].

Current research demonstrates the nascent promise of autonomous soft-tissue robots. However, more advances are required to bring new AI technologies efficiently into play in computer-assisted neurosurgery.

3   Internet of Things (IoT) in Neurosurgery

3.1   The Concept of IoT

IoT, Internet of Things, is defined as a networked interconnection of objects. It represents a self-configuring wireless network of sensors made to interconnect all things. A thing or object is any item that can join a communication chain. Since the primary purpose of IoT is to offer communication capabilities characterized by data transmission, a communication module such as a radio-frequency identification (RFID) or Bluetooth module is its main constituent [92]. Such modules are embedded in complex systems using sensors to collect information from their environment for continually tracking and accounting for millions of things [93].

3.2   IoT Applications in Neurology and Neurosurgery

Today, IoT technology is widely applied in health care, the so-called internet of medical things. This can be imagined as a building of a infrastructure of software applications that connect medical staff, patients, wearable devices, information technology systems, and medical devices, to collect more precise, relevant, and high-quality data and incorporate all of them in real time [94, 95]. Such technology provides promising potential benefits by monitoring processes and outcomes, which in turn increases workforce productivity, saves costs [96], improves operational efficiency [97], enhances patient care and safety, and minimizes human errors [98, 99]. In neurology, many IoT-based systems have been applied including a fall-risk prediction system for gait patients [100–102], wearables for behavior analysis and neurological rehabilitation in Parkinson's disease [54, 103–106], wearables for sleep monitoring [92, 107–113], seizure prediction [114–117], early detection and monitoring systems for Alzheimer disease [103, 118–120], rehabilitation systems for dementia and stroke [121–124], wearable EEGs to monitor different neurological states [125–128], and systems that analyze a patient's functional status to assess postoperative surgical outcomes in degenerative spinal disease [14, 129].

3.2.1   Operating Room-Related Applications
More related to the surgical operating theater, despite the considerable lag in IoT-based advancement, IoT can first be used in the sterilization process. Control of surgical infection through improving the sterilization of surgical instruments is important for lowering costs and improving safety and effectiveness in medical institutions [130], using wireless temperature sensors with systems to monitor for sterilization error, validity, and safety stock calculation [131]. IoT sensing

technology can be applied through: a Pack Sterilization Error Alarm Interface, which helps to achieve instant notification and handling when an error occurs according to the sterilization standard; a Pack Expiration Alarm Interface, showing whether the pack has expired or will soon do so; and the Insufficient Stock Alarm Interface, reporting any shortage of the stock of packs according to their sterilization state, showing the exact number of packs that need to be sterilized, and the quantity needed to supply the pack requirements [131]. Therefore, besides ensuring the safety of the sterilization process and lowering costs, devices to monitor the different sterilization items and the effect of sterilization on them can enable us to detect problems in real time, analyze the causes, and propose methods for improvement. By those means we can control hospital infections effectively.

Moreover, an IoT-driven system was used to visualize the movements of surgical instruments during procedures, including the surgeon's forceps and electrocautery probe. This provided live feedback from each device to the surgeon on a PC screen. Thus, this technique enables the factors affecting surgical performance to be studied, which in turn enhances surgical performance and ensures patient safety [132].

Furthermore, Nexeon MedSystems has invented a deep brain stimulation (DBS) device that can record the local field potentials of neuronal activity, and extract, analyze, and use such recordings to produce self-adjusting algorithms. Thus, the stimulus and the collected signals would enable therapy for movement disorders to be automatically optimized. It can also be correlated with the patient's external state or information about actions, offering more advanced insights into the way in which a given illness affects a patient. The same company has created the CranialSuite system, which is a surgical planning tool combining basic trajectory planning with innovative planning and navigation competences to obtain frame settings, which improve surgical theater workflow and locate anatomical and functional areas precisely. It has also created the CranialCloud framework, which connects directly recorded signals from the patient's brain with surgical images from planning systems to retrieve lead brain locations and patients' post-therapeutic responses [133].

More advanced is the ability to combine IoT, big data technologies, and cloud computing in real time. With information and communication technology, this has enabled IoT devices to act as sensory inputs to robots. Thus, medical robots as previously described have found significant applications in patient monitoring, surgery, prosthetic robotics for amputated legs or arms, and for patients with muscle disorders or cognitive or mental disabilities. The prosthetic robotic limb identifies the patient's intention and controls its movement by sensing muscle pressure and the related nerves via the sensors attached to the amputated area. Likewise, in the operation room, an IoT-driven camera can provide visual sensory inputs and analyze the field, together with the data retrieved through monitoring the patient, to inform the robot how to perform a surgery [134]. Furthermore, RFID tags can be implemented in surgical instruments so they are easily identified and automatically recognized [135]. An antenna system has been developed to detect the RFID tags, so each surgical instrument in the operating room can be traced [136]. Similarly, through digitalization of the surgical scenario, medical staff motion and the workflow can be automatically detected and analyzed in real time during surgery [137]. The OPeLiNK system has been developed similarly, and it was through this that SCOT, a system that interconnects medical devices, was invented [18].

4   The Smart Cyber Operating Theater (SCOT)

An intelligent operating room has been developed that enables navigation to be updated intraoperatively using MRI brain images, measures evoked potentials to monitor brain function, and provides rapid diagnosis support [138–142]. Thus, it helps to avoid brain shift, provides the ability to check for residual tumors before the end of surgery, and achieves higher survival rates through repeatedly obtained biological information from various items of equipment that provide feedback between intraoperative analysis and treatment [143]. However, in an intelligent operating room, the surgeon is the one who has to integrate the different kinds of information obtained from each device to make an informed decision, which is called an information-guided surgery or a basic SCOT. Hence, to integrate all the information fully, the standard SCOT was invented [18]. The core component of the standard SCOT, in addition to the open MRI and the rapid diagnostic test systems, is the communication interface, which is used to connect and network all devices in the operating environment. Okamoto et al. developed a new operating room interface, the OPeLiNK [18], based on the ORiN, the Open Resource interface for the Network, widely used in industry [144–146]. Decision making, especially during malignant tumor surgeries, depends not only on MRI-acquired morphological data or the navigation system, but also on functional data such as cerebral cortex location, in addition to histological data of the indicated cell malignancy. Therefore, implementation of the cyber-physical system in the operating room, the SCOT, would develop the function of information presentation and help in making decisions during an operation. It allows heterogeneous data including cautery knife power, positional data about the surgical instruments, evoked potential test records, patient monitoring data, anesthetic data, intraoperative imaging findings, the neuro-navigation system, and the surgical field video data to be integrated in real time [17]. In addition, it enables an optimal layout of the several forms of data, collected as numerical data except for the imaging data, to be designed. All these data can then be displayed on a surgical strategy desk for the surgeon and staff in the surgical operating room, and even in a supervising doctor's office, in real time (Figs. 8 and 9) [18]. As a result, information can be evaluated in the same timeline, allowing efficient discussion and decision making to ensue. Furthermore, these collected data can be recorded and compared with the time synchronization to detect any complication caused by the operation, thus improving the transparency of the surgery. Moreover, it can help in developing a database by recording postoperative recurrence rates and complication data, and automatically refer the morphological idiosyncracies of each patient to a standard brain form, which enables past and current treatments to be compared [18].

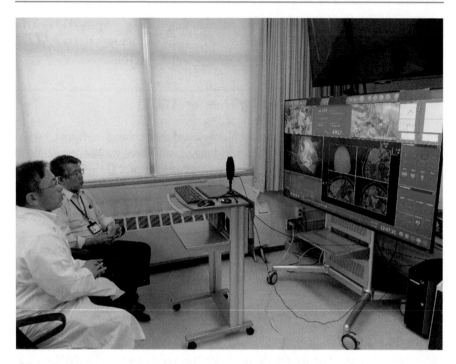

Fig. 8 Strategy desk; the monitor information system is in a separate room from the operation room. The commander surgeon judges the performance of the surgery and determines the next procedure

The greatest implementation that can be applied in image-guided procedures is achieving precision, through the integration of image and positional information from intraoperative modalities, surgical navigation systems, and a positioned robot in middleware. In addition, since equipment robotization makes it possible to automate the surgical environment, the operating room can be set for each surgical case pattern by the development of a robotic operating table or a robotic surgical microscope. This setting reduces the preparation time for operations, and also makes it possible to move the patient automatically using the robotic operating table. The application of a decision making navigation system along with robotized equipment is called a Hyper SCOT [18].

To date, SCOT has been used for a successful and complete resection of a pituitary adenoma via an endoscopic endonasal approach at Shinshu University Hospital [17]. More recently, the three types of SCOT, Basic, Standard, and Hyper SCOT have been applied by Muragaki et al. in Tokyo Women's Medical University for 56 cases of brain tumors and functional and orthopedic diseases; the outcome results are not yet published [147].

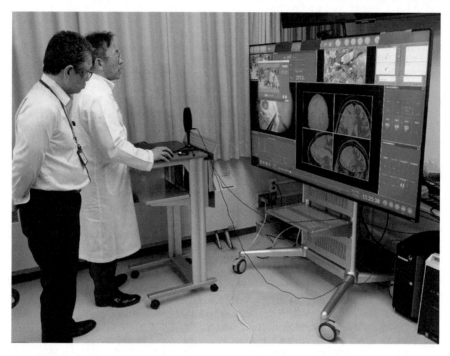

Fig. 9 The commander surgeon and the operator can call each other. Messages can be shared not only verbally but also as drawings on the monitor

5   Conclusion and Future Directions

Diagnosis, treatment, and monitoring of patients using AI and medical IoT have entered the clinical phase in neurosurgery, despite limited interest from many neurosurgeons. Understanding of clinically applicable AI-driven automated surgical robots will augment surgical capability to enhance outcomes and permit better access to care. Thanks to the continuing progress of networks, sensors, and AI-facilitated automation technology, the diversity and accuracy of medical IoT have been improved. It is feasible to build a smart operating room, the SCOT, to be used in either microscopic or endoscopic neurosurgery. Such technology will help exploit the most appropriate usage of surgical instruments, improve the safety of surgical procedures and standardize them, and enhance the quality of surgical treatment overall. However, many applications remain in the validation phase, as AI research involving medical IoT in neurosurgery is still in its infancy. Therefore, it merits further research. In addition, if neurosurgeons understand the basic concepts and possibilities of AI and IoT applications, this could lead to a paradigm shift in diagnosis and treatment of neurosurgical diseases.

References

1. Yoon D. What we need to prepare for the fourth industrial revolution. Healthc Inform Res. 2017;23:75. https://doi.org/10.4258/hir.2017.23.2.75.
2. National Academies of Sciences, Engineering, and Medicine. The fourth industrial revolution: proceedings of a workshop–in brief. The National Academies Press; 2017. https://doi. org/10.17226/24699.
3. Obermeyer Z, Emanuel EJ. Predicting the future — big data, machine learning, and clinical medicine. N Engl J Med. 2016;375(13):1216–9. https://doi.org/10.1056/NEJMp1606181.
4. Jordan MI, Mitchell TM. Machine learning: trends, perspectives, and prospects. Science (80-). 2015;349(6245):255–60. https://doi.org/10.1126/science.aaa8415.
5. Fomenko A, Lozano A. Artificial intelligence in neurosurgery. Univ Tor Med J. 2019;96:19–21.
6. Senders J, Arnaout O, Karhade A, et al. Natural and artificial intelligence in neurosurgery: a systematic review. Neurosurgery. 2017;83:181–92. https://doi.org/10.1093/ neuros/nyx384.
7. Ahmed Z, Mohamed K, Zeeshan S, Dong X. Artificial intelligence with multi-functional machine learning platform development for better healthcare and precision medicine. Database J Biol Databases Curat. 2020;2020:baaa010. https://doi.org/10.1093/database/ baaa010.
8. Galbusera F, Casaroli G, Bassani T. Artificial intelligence and machine learning in spine research. Jor Spine. 2019;2(1):e1044. https://doi.org/10.1002/jsp2.1044.
9. Hoy M. The "Internet of Things": what it is and what it means for libraries. Med Ref Serv Q. 2015;34:353–8. https://doi.org/10.1080/02763869.2015.1052699.
10. Nam K, Kim D, Choi B, Han I. Internet of Things, digital biomarker, and artificial intelligence in spine: current and future perspectives. Neurospine. 2019;16:705–11. https://doi. org/10.14245/ns.1938388.194.
11. Hoeks L, de Ranitz-Greven W, de Valk H. Real-time continuous glucose monitoring system for treatment of diabetes: a systematic review. Diabet Med. 2011;28:386–94. https://doi. org/10.1111/j.1464-5491.2010.03177.x.
12. Rumpler M, Mader JK, Fischer JP, et al. First application of a transcutaneous optical single-port glucose monitoring device in patients with type 1 diabetes mellitus. Biosens Bioelectron. 2017;88:240–8. https://doi.org/10.1016/j.bios.2016.08.039.
13. Mora H, Gil D, Terol R, Azorin-Lopez J, Szymanski J. An IoT-based computational framework for healthcare monitoring in mobile environments. Sensors. 2017;17:2302. https://doi. org/10.3390/s17102302.
14. Chakravorty A, Mobbs R, Anderson D, et al. The role of wearable devices and objective gait analysis for the assessment and monitoring of patients with lumbar spinal stenosis: systematic review. BMC Musculoskelet Disord. 2019;20 https://doi.org/10.1186/s12891-019-2663-4.
15. Meinert E, Van Velthoven M, Brindley D, et al. The Internet of Things in health care in Oxford: protocol for proof-of-concept projects. JMIR Res Protoc. 2018;7(12):e12077. https://doi.org/10.2196/12077.
16. Rajiv. What are the major components of Internet of Things. Published 2018. https://www. rfpage.com/what-are-the-major-components-of-internet-of-things/
17. Nakamura T, Ogiwara T, Goto T, et al. Clinical experience of endoscopic endonasal approach in the innovative, newly developed operating room "smart cyber operating theater (SCOT)". World Neurosurg. 2020;134:293–6. https://doi.org/10.1016/j.wneu.2019.11.021.
18. Okamoto J, Masamune K, Iseki H, Muragaki Y. Development concepts of a Smart Cyber Operating Theater (SCOT) using ORiN technology. Biomed Eng/Biomed Tech. 2017;63:31–7. https://doi.org/10.1515/bmt-2017-0006.
19. Ghahramani Z. Probabilistic machine learning and artificial intelligence. Nature. 2015;521(7553):452–9. https://doi.org/10.1038/nature14541.

20. Senders JT, Arnaout O, Karhade AV, et al. Natural and artificial intelligence in neurosurgery: a systematic review. Neurosurgery. 2018;83(2):181–92. https://doi.org/10.1093/neuros/nyx384.
21. Rajpurkar P, Irvin J, Zhu K, et al. CheXNet: radiologist-level pneumonia detection on chest X-Rays with deep learning. Published online November 14, 2017.
22. Esteva A, Kuprel B, Novoa RA, et al. Dermatologist-level classification of skin cancer with deep neural networks. Nature. 2017;542(7639):115–8. https://doi.org/10.1038/nature21056.
23. He J, Baxter SL, Xu J, Xu J, Zhou X, Zhang K. The practical implementation of artificial intelligence technologies in medicine. Nat Med. 2019;25(1):30–6. https://doi.org/10.1038/s41591-018-0307-0.
24. Titano JJ, Badgeley M, Schefflein J, et al. Automated deep-neural-network surveillance of cranial images for acute neurologic events. Nat Med. 2018;24(9):1337–41. https://doi.org/10.1038/s41591-018-0147-y.
25. Bennett CC, Hauser K. Artificial intelligence framework for simulating clinical decision-making: a Markov decision process approach. Artif Intell Med. 2013;57(1):9–19. https://doi.org/10.1016/j.artmed.2012.12.003.
26. Volkov M, Hashimoto DA, Rosman G, Meireles OR, Rus D. Machine learning and coresets for automated real-time video segmentation of laparoscopic and robot-assisted surgery. In: 2017 IEEE international conference on robotics and automation (ICRA); 2017. p. 754–9. https://doi.org/10.1109/ICRA.2017.7989093.
27. Stauder R, Okur A, Peter L, et al. Random forests for phase detection in surgical workflow analysis. In: Stoyanov D, Collins DL, Sakuma I, Abolmaesumi P, Jannin P, editors. BT - information processing in computer-assisted interventions. Springer; 2014. p. 148–57.
28. Burns JE, Yao J, Summers RM. Vertebral body compression fractures and bone density: automated detection and classification on CT images. Radiology. 2017;284(3):788–97. https://doi.org/10.1148/radiol.2017162100.
29. Ueda D, Yamamoto A, Nishimori M, et al. Deep learning for MR angiography: automated detection of cerebral aneurysms. Radiology. 2018;290(1):187–94. https://doi.org/10.1148/radiol.2018180901.
30. Topol EJ. High-performance medicine: the convergence of human and artificial intelligence. Nat Med. 2019;25(1):44–56. https://doi.org/10.1038/s41591-018-0300-7.
31. Rajkomar A, Dean J, Kohane I. Machine learning in medicine. N Engl J Med. 2019;380(14):1347–58. https://doi.org/10.1056/NEJMra1814259.
32. Panesar S, Cagle Y, Chander D, Morey J, Fernandez-Miranda J, Kliot M. Artificial intelligence and the future of surgical robotics. Ann Surg. 2019;270(2):223–6. https://journals.lww.com/annalsofsurgery/Fulltext/2019/08000/Artificial_Intelligence_and_the_Future_of_Surgical.7.aspx
33. Bohl MA, Oppenlander ME, Spetzler R. A prospective cohort evaluation of a robotic, auto-navigating operating microscope. Cureus. 2016;8(6):e662. https://doi.org/10.7759/cureus.662.
34. Surgical robotics. Evaluation of the computer motion AESOP 3000 robotic endoscope holder. Health Devices. 2002;31(7):256–68.
35. Yu J, Shi Z, Lian Y, et al. Noninvasive IDH1 mutation estimation based on a quantitative radiomics approach for grade II glioma. Eur Radiol. 2017;27(8):3509–22. https://doi.org/10.1007/s00330-016-4653-3.
36. Ahn SS, Shin N-Y, Chang JH, et al. Prediction of methylguanine methyltransferase promoter methylation in glioblastoma using dynamic contrast-enhanced magnetic resonance and diffusion tensor imaging. J Neurosurg JNS. 2014;121(2):367–73. https://doi.org/10.3171/2014.5.JNS132279.
37. Kickingereder P, Bonekamp D, Nowosielski M, et al. Radiogenomics of glioblastoma: machine learning-based classification of molecular characteristics by using multiparametric and multiregional MR imaging features. Radiology. 2016;281:161382. https://doi.org/10.1148/radiol.2016161382.

38. Panesar SS, D'Souza RN, Yeh F-C, Fernandez-Miranda JC. Machine learning versus logistic regression methods for 2-year mortality prognostication in a small, heterogeneous glioma database. World Neurosurg X. 2019;2:100012. https://doi.org/10.1016/j.wnsx.2019.100012.

39. Chang K, Bai HX, Zhou H, et al. Residual convolutional neural network for the determination of *IDH* status in low- and high-grade gliomas from MR imaging. Clin Cancer Res. 2018;24(5):1073–81. https://doi.org/10.1158/1078-0432.CCR-17-2236.

40. Panesar S, Kliot M, Parrish R, Fernandez-Miranda J, Cagle Y, Britz G. Promises and perils of artificial intelligence in neurosurgery. Neurosurgery. 2019;87:33–44. https://doi.org/10.1093/neuros/nyz471.

41. Brown AD, Marotta TR. Using machine learning for sequence-level automated MRI protocol selection in neuroradiology. J Am Med Informatics Assoc. 2018;25(5):568–71. https://doi.org/10.1093/jamia/ocx125.

42. Zhou H, Vallières M, Bai HX, et al. MRI features predict survival and molecular markers in diffuse lower-grade gliomas. Neuro-Oncology. 2017;19(6):862–70. https://doi.org/10.1093/neuonc/now256.

43. Kassahun Y, Perrone R, De Momi E, et al. Automatic classification of epilepsy types using ontology-based and genetics-based machine learning. Artif Intell Med. 2014;61(2):79–88. https://doi.org/10.1016/j.artmed.2014.03.001.

44. Zhang B, Chang K, Ramkissoon S, et al. Multimodal MRI features predict isocitrate dehydrogenase genotype in high-grade gliomas. Neuro-Oncology. 2017;19(1):109–17. https://doi.org/10.1093/neuonc/now121.

45. Chen R, Snyder M. Promise of personalized omics to precision medicine. Wiley Interdiscip Rev Syst Biol Med. 2013;5(1):73–82. https://doi.org/10.1002/wsbm.1198.

46. Fereidouni F, Harmany ZT, Tian M, et al. Microscopy with ultraviolet surface excitation for rapid slide-free histology. Nat Biomed Eng. 2017;1(12):957–66. https://doi.org/10.1038/s41551-017-0165-y.

47. Tankus A, Yeshurun Y, Fried I. An automatic measure for classifying clusters of suspected spikes into single cells versus multiunits. J Neural Eng. 2009;6(5):56001. https://doi.org/10.1088/1741-2560/6/5/056001.

48. Emblem KE, Nedregaard B, Hald JK, Nome T, Due-Tonnessen P, Bjornerud A. Automatic glioma characterization from dynamic susceptibility contrast imaging: brain tumor segmentation using knowledge-based fuzzy clustering. J Magn Reson Imaging. 2009;30(1):1–10. https://doi.org/10.1002/jmri.21815.

49. Emblem KE, Pinho MC, Zöllner FG, et al. A generic support vector machine model for preoperative glioma survival associations. Radiology. 2014;275(1):228–34. https://doi.org/10.1148/radiol.14140770.

50. Rughani A, Dumont T, Lu Z, et al. Use of an artificial neural network to predict head injury outcome: clinical article. J Neurosurg. 2009;113:585–90. https://doi.org/10.3171/2009.11.JNS09857.

51. Lee JS, Lee DS, Kim S-K, et al. Localization of epileptogenic zones in F-18 FDG brain PET of patients with temporal lobe epilepsy using artificial neural network. IEEE Trans Med Imaging. 2000;19(4):347–55. https://doi.org/10.1109/42.848185.

52. Kerr WT, Nguyen ST, Cho AY, et al. Computer-aided diagnosis and localization of lateralized temporal lobe epilepsy using interictal FDG-PET. Front Neurol. 2013;4:31. https://doi.org/10.3389/fneur.2013.00031.

53. Chiang S, Levin HS, Haneef Z. Computer-automated focus lateralization of temporal lobe epilepsy using fMRI. J Magn Reson Imaging. 2015;41(6):1689–94. https://doi.org/10.1002/jmri.24696.

54. Cohen KB, Glass B, Greiner HM, et al. Methodological issues in predicting pediatric epilepsy surgery candidates through natural language processing and machine learning. Biomed Inform Insights. 2016;8:11–8. https://doi.org/10.4137/BII.S38308.

55. Clarke LP, Velthuizen RP, Clark M, et al. MRI measurement of brain tumor response: comparison of visual metric and automatic segmentation. Magn Reson Imaging. 1998;16(3):271–9. https://doi.org/10.1016/S0730-725X(97)00302-0.

56. Dolz J, Betrouni N, Quidet M, et al. Stacking denoising auto-encoders in a deep network to segment the brainstem on MRI in brain cancer patients: a clinical study. Comput Med Imaging Graph. 2016;52:8–18. https://doi.org/10.1016/j.compmedimag.2016.03.003.

57. Dumont T, Rughani A, Tranmer B. Prediction of symptomatic cerebral vasospasm after aneurysmal subarachnoid hemorrhage with an artificial neural network: feasibility and comparison with logistic regression models. World Neurosurg. 2011;75:57–63.; discussion 25. https://doi.org/10.1016/j.wneu.2010.07.007.

58. Anne N, Bo HM, Anna T, Kim M. Prediction of tissue outcome and assessment of treatment effect in acute ischemic stroke using deep learning. Stroke. 2018;49(6):1394–401. https://doi.org/10.1161/STROKEAHA.117.019740.

59. Kitajima M, Hirai T, Katsuragawa S, et al. Differentiation of common large sellar-suprasellar masses. Effect of artificial neural network on radiologists' diagnosis performance. Acad Radiol. 2009;16:313–20. https://doi.org/10.1016/j.acra.2008.09.015.

60. C. DR. Machine learning in medicine. Circulation. 2015;132(20):1920–30. https://doi.org/10.1161/CIRCULATIONAHA.115.001593.

61. Rolston JD, Zygourakis CC, Han SJ, Lau CY, Berger MS, Parsa AT. Medical errors in neurosurgery. Surg Neurol Int. 2014;5(Suppl 10):S435–40. https://doi.org/10.4103/2152-7806.142777.

62. Weede O, Mönnich H, Müller B, Wörn H. An intelligent and autonomous endoscopic guidance system for minimally invasive surgery. In: 2011 IEEE international conference on robotics and automation; 2011. p. 5762–8. https://doi.org/10.1109/ICRA.2011.5980216.

63. Pandya S, Motkoski J, Serrano-Almeida C, Greer A, Latour I, Sutherland G. Advancing neurosurgery with image-guided robotics technical note. J Neurosurg. 2009;111:1141–9. https://doi.org/10.3171/2009.2.JNS081334.

64. D'Albis T, Haegelen C, Essert C, Fernández-Vidal S, Lalys F, Jannin P. PyDBS: an automated image processing workflow for deep brain stimulation surgery. Int J Comput Assist Radiol Surg. 2015;10(2):117–28. https://doi.org/10.1007/s11548-014-1007-y.

65. Li Q. Computer-assisted neurosurgery: yesterday, today and tomorrow. Published online August 23, 2017.

66. Girão PS, Ramos PMP, Postolache O, Miguel Dias Pereira J. Tactile sensors for robotic applications. Measurement. 2013;46(3):1257–71. https://doi.org/10.1016/j.measurement.2012.11.015.

67. Tzou H, Lee H-J, Arnold S. Smart materials, precision sensors/actuators, smart structures, and structronic systems. Mech Adv Mater Struct. 2004;11:367–93. https://doi.org/10.1080/15376490490451552.

68. Shademan A, Decker RS, Opfermann JD, Leonard S, Krieger A, Kim PCW. Supervised autonomous robotic soft tissue surgery. Sci Transl Med. 2016;8(337):337ra64. https://doi.org/10.1126/scitranslmed.aad9398.

69. Camarillo DB, Krummel TM, Salisbury JK. Robotic technology in surgery: past, present, and future. Am J Surg. 2004;188(4A Suppl):2–15. https://doi.org/10.1016/j.amjsurg.2004.08.025.

70. Kwoh YS, Hou J, Jonckheere EA, Hayati S. A robot with improved absolute positioning accuracy for CT guided stereotactic brain surgery. IEEE Trans Biomed Eng. 1988;35(2):153–60. https://doi.org/10.1109/10.1354.

71. Grimm F, Naros G, Gutenberg A, Keric N, Giese A, Gharabaghi A. Blurring the boundaries between frame-based and frameless stereotaxy: feasibility study for brain biopsies performed with the use of a head-mounted robot. J Neurosurg JNS. 2015;123(3):737–42. https://doi.org/10.3171/2014.12.JNS141781.

72. Gonzalez-Martinez J, Vadera S, Mullin J, et al. Robot-assisted stereotactic laser ablation in medically intractable epilepsy: operative technique. Neurosurgery. 2014;10(Suppl 2):163–7. https://doi.org/10.1227/neu.0000000000000286.

73. Dorfer C, Minchev G, Czech T, et al. A novel miniature robotic device for frameless implantation of depth electrodes in refractory epilepsy. J Neurosurg JNS. 2016;126(5):1622–8. https://doi.org/10.3171/2016.5.JNS16388.

74. Li QH, Zamorano L, Pandya A, Perez R, Gong J, Diaz F. The application accuracy of the neuromate robot—a quantitative comparison with frameless and frame-based surgical localization systems. Comput Aided Surg. 2002;7(2):90–8. https://doi.org/10.3109/10929080209146020.

75. Ahmed SI, Javed G, Mubeen B, et al. Robotics in neurosurgery: a literature review. J Pak Med Assoc. 2018;68(2):258–63.
76. Haegelen C, Touzet G, Reyns N, Maurage C-A, Ayachi M, Blond S. Stereotactic robot-guided biopsies of brain stem lesions: experience with 15 cases. Neurochirurgie. 2010;56(5):363–7. https://doi.org/10.1016/j.neuchi.2010.05.006.
77. Amin DV, Lunsford LD. Volumetric resection using the surgiScope®: a quantitative accuracy analysis of robot-assisted resection. Stereotact Funct Neurosurg. 2004;82(5–6):250–3. https://doi.org/10.1159/000083177.
78. Vadera S, Chan A, Lo T, et al. Frameless stereotactic robot-assisted subthalamic nucleus deep brain stimulation: case report. World Neurosurg. 2015;97:762.e11–4. https://doi.org/10.1016/j.wneu.2015.11.009.
79. Hu X, Ohnmeiss DD, Lieberman IH. Robotic-assisted pedicle screw placement: lessons learned from the first 102 patients. Eur Spine J. 2013;22(3):661–6. https://doi.org/10.1007/s00586-012-2499-1.
80. Nathoo N, Cavuşoğlu M, Vogelbaum M, Barnett G. In touch with robotics: neurosurgery for the future. Neurosurgery. 2005;56:421–33.; discussion 421. https://doi.org/10.1227/01.NEU.0000153929.68024.CF.
81. Leonard S, Wu KL, Kim Y, Krieger A, Kim PCW. Smart tissue anastomosis robot (STAR): a vision-guided robotics system for laparoscopic suturing. IEEE Trans Biomed Eng. 2014;61(4):1305–17. https://doi.org/10.1109/TBME.2014.2302385.
82. Kassahun Y, Yu B, Tibebu A, et al. Surgical robotics beyond enhanced dexterity instrumentation: a survey of machine learning techniques and their role in intelligent and autonomous surgical actions. Int J Comput Assist Radiol Surg. 2015;11:553–68. https://doi.org/10.1007/s11548-015-1305-z.
83. Huang H-M. The autonomy levels for unmanned systems (ALFUS) framework interim results. Published online January 1, 2006.
84. Yip M, Das N. Robot autonomy for surgery. Published Online July 10, 2017.
85. Lin HC, Shafran I, Murphy TE, Okamura AM, Yuh DD, Hager GD. Automatic detection and segmentation of robot-assisted surgical motions. In: Duncan JS, Gerig G, editors. BT - medical image computing and computer-assisted intervention – MICCAI 2005. Berlin Heidelberg: Springer; 2005. p. 802–10.
86. Murali A, Garg A, Krishnan S, et al. TSC-DL: unsupervised trajectory segmentation of multi-modal surgical demonstrations with Deep Learning. In: 2016 IEEE international conference on robotics and automation (ICRA); 2016. p. 4150–7. https://doi.org/10.1109/ICRA.2016.7487607.
87. Gao Y, Vedula S, Reiley CE, et al. JHU-ISI gesture and skill assessment working set (JIGSAWS): a surgical activity dataset for human motion modeling. 2014.
88. Cavusoglu MC, Tendick F, Cohn M, Sastry SS. A laparoscopic telesurgical workstation. IEEE Trans Robot Autom. 1999;15(4):728–39. https://doi.org/10.1109/70.782027.
89. Mayer H, Gomez F, Wierstra D, Nagy I, Knoll A, Schmidhuber J. A system for robotic heart surgery that learns to tie knots using recurrent neural networks. In: 2006 IEEE/RSJ international conference on intelligent robots and systems; 2006. p. 543–8. https://doi.org/10.1109/IROS.2006.282190.
90. Murali A, Sen S, Kehoe B, et al. Learning by observation for surgical subtasks: multilateral cutting of 3D viscoelastic and 2D orthotropic tissue phantoms. In: 2015 IEEE international conference on robotics and automation (ICRA); 2015. p. 1202–9. https://doi.org/10.1109/ICRA.2015.7139344.
91. Adler JR Jr, Chang SD, Murphy MJ, Doty J, Geis P, Hancock SL. The Cyberknife: a frameless robotic system for radiosurgery. Stereotact Funct Neurosurg. 1997;69(1–4):124–8. https://doi.org/10.1159/000099863.
92. Gubbi J, Buyya R, Marusic S, Palaniswami M. Internet of Things (IoT): a vision, architectural elements, and future directions. Futur Gener Comput Syst. 2013;29(7):1645–60. https://doi.org/10.1016/j.future.2013.01.010.

93. Möller DPF. Introduction to the Internet of Things. In: Möller DPF, editor. BT - guide to computing fundamentals in cyber-physical systems: concepts, design methods, and applications. Springer; 2016. p. 141–84. https://doi.org/10.1007/978-3-319-25178-3_4.

94. Gupta PK, Maharaj BT, Malekian R. A novel and secure IoT based cloud centric architecture to perform predictive analysis of users activities in sustainable health centres. Multimed Tools Appl. 2017;76(18):18489–512. https://doi.org/10.1007/s11042-016-4050-6.

95. Kamalanathan N, Eardley A, Chibelushi C, Collins T. Improving the patient discharge planning process through knowledge management by using the Internet of Things. Adv Internet Things. 2013;03:16–26. https://doi.org/10.4236/ait.2013.32A003.

96. Riggins FJ, Wamba SF. Research directions on the adoption, usage, and impact of the Internet of Things through the use of big data analytics. In: 2015 48th Hawaii international conference on system sciences; 2015. p. 1531–40. https://doi.org/10.1109/HICSS.2015.186.

97. Alsmirat MA, Jararweh Y, Obaidat I, Gupta BB. Internet of surveillance: a cloud supported large-scale wireless surveillance system. J Supercomput. 2017;73(3):973–92. https://doi.org/10.1007/s11227-016-1857-x.

98. Joyia G, Liaqat R, Farooq A, Rehman S. Internet of medical things (IOMT): applications, benefits and future challenges in healthcare domain. J Commun. 2017;12:240–7. https://doi.org/10.12720/jcm.12.4.240-247.

99. Qi J, Yang P, Min G, Amft O, Dong F, Xu L. Advanced Internet of Things for personalised healthcare systems: a survey. Pervasive Mob Comput. 2017;41:132–49. https://doi.org/10.1016/j.pmcj.2017.06.018.

100. van Schooten KS, Pijnappels M, Rispens SM, Elders PJM, Lips P, van Dieën JH. Ambulatory fall-risk assessment: amount and quality of daily-life gait predict falls in older adults. J Gerontol Ser A. 2015;70(5):608–15. https://doi.org/10.1093/gerona/glu225.

101. Schwenk M, Hauer K, Zieschang T, Englert S, Mohler J, Najafi B. Sensor-derived physical activity parameters can predict future falls in people with dementia. Gerontology. 2014;60(6):483–92. https://doi.org/10.1159/000363136.

102. Abtahi M, Gyllinsky JV, Paesang B, et al. MagicSox: an E-textile IoT system to quantify gait abnormalities. Smart Heal. 2018;5-6:4–14. https://doi.org/10.1016/j.smhl.2017.10.002.

103. Alvarez F, Popa M, Solachidis V, et al. Behavior analysis through multimodal sensing for care of Parkinson's and Alzheimer's patients. IEEE Multimed. 2018;25(1):14–25. https://doi.org/10.1109/MMUL.2018.011921232.

104. Memedi M, Tshering G, Fogelberg M, Jusufi I, Kolkowska E, Klein G. An interface for IoT: feeding back health-related data to Parkinson's disease patients. J Sens Actuator Netw. 2018;7(1):14. https://doi.org/10.3390/jsan7010014.

105. Kim D, Hwang S, Kim M, Song JH, Lee S-W, Kim IK. Development of Parkinson patient generated data collection platform using FHIR and IoT devices. Stud Health Technol Inform. 2017;245:141–5.

106. Giuberti M, Ferrari G, Contin L, et al. Assigning UPDRS scores in the leg agility task of parkinsonians: can it be done through BSN-based kinematic variables? IEEE Internet Things J. 2015;2(1):41–51. https://doi.org/10.1109/JIOT.2015.2390075.

107. Shah SA, Ren A, Fan D, et al. Internet of Things for sensing: a case study in the healthcare system. Appl Sci. 2018;8(4):508. https://doi.org/10.3390/app8040508.

108. Lin C, Prasad M, Chung C, et al. IoT-based wireless polysomnography intelligent system for sleep monitoring. IEEE Access. 2018;6:405–14. https://doi.org/10.1109/ACCESS.2017.2765702.

109. Yacchirema D, Sarabia-Jácome D, Palau CE, Esteve M. System for monitoring and supporting the treatment of sleep apnea using IoT and big data. Pervasive Mob Comput. 2018;50:25–40. https://doi.org/10.1016/j.pmcj.2018.07.007.

110. Choi JH, Kang UG, Lee BM. Sleep information gathering protocol using CoAP for sleep care. Entropy. 2017;19(9):450. https://doi.org/10.3390/e19090450.

111. Liu J, Chen Y, Wang Y, Chen X, Cheng J, Yang J. Monitoring vital signs and postures during sleep using WiFi signals. IEEE Internet Things J. 2018;5(3):2071–84. https://doi.org/10.1109/JIOT.2018.2822818.

112. Surrel G, Aminifar A, Rincón F, Murali S, Atienza D. Online obstructive sleep apnea detection on medical wearable sensors. IEEE Trans Biomed Circuits Syst. 2018;12(4):762–73. https://doi.org/10.1109/TBCAS.2018.2824659.
113. Swangarom S, Tajima T, Abe T, Kimura H. A proposal for a sleep disorder detection system. Sensors Mater. 2018;30:1457. https://doi.org/10.18494/SAM.2018.1882.
114. Vergara PM, de la Cal E, Villar JR, González VM, Sedano J. An IoT platform for epilepsy monitoring and supervising. J Sensors. 2017;2017:6043069. https://doi.org/10.1155/2017/6043069.
115. Alhussein M, Muhammad G, Hossain MS, Amin SU. Cognitive IoT-cloud integration for smart healthcare: case study for epileptic seizure detection and monitoring. Mob Netw Appl. 2018;23(6):1624–35. https://doi.org/10.1007/s11036-018-1113-0.
116. Lin S-K, Istiqomah, Wang L-C, Lin C-Y, Chiueh H. An ultra-low power smart headband for real-time epileptic seizure detection. IEEE J Transl Eng Heal Med. 2018;6:1–10. https://doi.org/10.1109/JTEHM.2018.2861882.
117. Hosseini M, Pompili D, Elisevich K, Soltanian-Zadeh H. Optimized deep learning for EEG big data and seizure prediction BCI via Internet of Things. IEEE Trans Big Data. 2017;3(4):392–404. https://doi.org/10.1109/TBDATA.2017.2769670.
118. Martinez de Lizarduy U, Calvo Salomón P, Gómez Vilda P, Ecay Torres M, López de Ipiña K. ALZUMERIC: a decision support system for diagnosis and monitoring of cognitive impairment. Loquens. 2017;4(1):e037. https://doi.org/10.3989/loquens.2017.037.
119. Varatharajan R, Manogaran G, Priyan MK, Sundarasekar R. Wearable sensor devices for early detection of Alzheimer disease using dynamic time warping algorithm. Cluster Comput. 2018;21(1):681–90. https://doi.org/10.1007/s10586-017-0977-2.
120. Yang G, Deng J, Pang G, et al. An IoT-enabled stroke rehabilitation system based on smart wearable armband and machine learning. IEEE J Transl Eng Heal Med. 2018;6:1–10. https://doi.org/10.1109/JTEHM.2018.2822681.
121. Rostill H, Nilforooshan R, Morgan A, Barnaghi P, Ream E, Chrysanthaki T. Technology integrated health management for dementia. Br J Community Nurs. 2018;23(10):502–8. https://doi.org/10.12968/bjcn.2018.23.10.502.
122. Atee M, Hoti K, Hughes JD. A technical note on the PainChek™ system: a web portal and mobile medical device for assessing pain in people with dementia. Front Aging Neurosci. 2018;10:117. https://www.frontiersin.org/article/10.3389/fnagi.2018.00117
123. Hoshino Y, Mitani K. A proposal of a usability scale system for rehabilitation games based on the cognitive therapeutic exercise. Int J Innov Comput Inf Control. 2018;14:1189–205. https://doi.org/10.24507/ijicic.14.04.1189.
124. Johansen B, Petersen MK, Korzepa MJ, Larsen J, Pontoppidan NH, Larsen JE. Personalizing the fitting of hearing aids by learning contextual preferences from Internet of Things data. Computers. 2018;7(1):1. https://doi.org/10.3390/computers7010001.
125. Mahajan R, Morshed BI, Bidelman GM. Design and validation of a wearable "DRL-less" EEG using a novel fully-reconfigurable architecture. In: 2016 38th annual international conference of the IEEE engineering in medicine and biology society (EMBC); 2016. p. 4999–5002. https://doi.org/10.1109/EMBC.2016.7591850.
126. Billeci L, Tonacci A, Tartarisco G, et al. An integrated approach for the monitoring of brain and autonomic response of children with autism spectrum disorders during treatment by wearable technologies. Front Neurosci. 2016;10:276. https://www.frontiersin.org/article/10.3389/fnins.2016.00276
127. Pinho F, Cerqueira J, Correia J, Sousa N, Dias N. myBrain: a novel EEG embedded system for epilepsy monitoring. J Med Eng Technol. 2017;41(7):564–85. https://doi.org/10.1080/03091902.2017.1382585.
128. Kassab A, Le Lan J, Tremblay J, et al. Multichannel wearable fNIRS-EEG system for long-term clinical monitoring: multichannel Wearable fNIRS-EEG System. Hum Brain Mapp. 2018;39:7–23. https://doi.org/10.1002/hbm.23849.
129. Kim DH, Nam KH, Choi BK, Han IH, Jeon TJ, Park SY. The usefulness of a wearable device in daily physical activity monitoring for the hospitalized patients undergoing lumbar surgery. J Korean Neurosurg Soc. 2019;62(5):561–6. https://doi.org/10.3340/jkns.2018.0131.

130. Mohapatra S. Sterilization and disinfection. In: Essentials of neuroanesthesia. Elsevier; 2017. p. 929–44.
131. Hung L-P, Peng C-J, Chen C-L. Using Internet of Things technology to improve patient safety in surgical instrument sterilization control. In: Chen J-L, Pang A-C, Deng D-J, Lin C-C, editors. BT - wireless internet. Springer; 2019. p. 183–92.
132. Ushimaru Y, Takahashi T, Souma Y, et al. Innovation in surgery/operating room driven by Internet of Things on medical devices. Surg Endosc. 2019;33:1–9. https://doi.org/10.1007/s00464-018-06651-4.
133. Rosellini W, D'Haese P-F. Data is driving the future of neurotechnology with cranialcloud. ONdrugDelivery. 2017;2017:44–7.
134. Patel AR, Patel RS, Singh NM, Kazi FS. Vitality of robotics in healthcare industry: an Internet of Things (IoT) perspective. In: Bhatt C, Dey N, Ashour AS, editors. BT - Internet of Things and big data technologies for next generation healthcare. Springer; 2017. p. 91–109. https://doi.org/10.1007/978-3-319-49736-5_5.
135. Yamashita K, Iwakami Y, Imaizumi K, et al. Identification of information surgical instrument by ceramic RFID tag. 2008 World Autom Congr WAC 2008. Published online January 1, 2008.
136. Kaori K, Kazuhiko Y, Akiko O, et al. Management of surgical instruments with radio frequency identification tags: a 27-month in hospital trial. Int J Health Care Qual Assur. 2016;29(2):236–47. https://doi.org/10.1108/IJHCQA-03-2015-0034.
137. Miyawaki F, Masamune K, Suzuki S, Yoshimitsu K, Vain J. Scrub nurse robot system-intraoperative motion analysis of a scrub nurse and timed-automata-based model for surgery. IEEE Trans Ind Electron. 2005;52(5):1227–35. https://doi.org/10.1109/TIE.2005.855692.
138. Iseki H, Muragaki Y, Nakamura R, et al. Intelligent operating theater using intraoperative open-MRI. Magn Reson Med Sci. 2005;4:129–36. https://doi.org/10.2463/mrms.4.129.
139. Iseki H, Nakamura R, Muragaki Y, et al. Advanced computer-aided intraoperative technologies for information-guided surgical management of gliomas: Tokyo women's medical university experience. Minim Invasive Neurosurg. 2008;51:285–91. https://doi.org/10.1055/s-0028-1082333.
140. Muragaki Y, Iseki H, Maruyama T, et al. Usefulness of intraoperative magnetic resonance imaging for glioma surgery. In: Nimsky C, Fahlbusch R, editors. BT - medical technologies in neurosurgery. Vienna: Springer; 2006. p. 67–75. https://doi.org/10.1007/978-3-211-33303-7_10.
141. Saito T, Muragaki Y, Maruyama T, et al. Difficulty in identification of the frontal language area in patients with dominant frontal gliomas that involve the pars triangularis. J Neurosurg. 2016;125:1–9. https://doi.org/10.3171/2015.8.JNS151204.
142. Shioyama T, Muragaki Y, Maruyama T, Komori T, Iseki H. Intraoperative flow cytometry analysis of glioma tissue for rapid determination of tumor presence and its histopathological grade: clinical article. J Neurosurg. 2013;118(6):1232–8.
143. Tamura M, Muragaki Y, Saito T, et al. Strategy of surgical resection for glioma based on intraoperative functional mapping and monitoring. Neurol Med Chir (Tokyo). 2015;55(5):383–98. https://doi.org/10.2176/nmc.ra.2014-0415.
144. Mizukawa M, Matsuka H, Koyama T, Matsumoto A. ORiN: open robot interface for the network, a proposed standard. Ind Robot An Int J. 2000;27:344–50. https://doi.org/10.1108/01439910010372992.
145. Mizukawa M, Matsuka H, Koyama T, et al. ORiN: open robot interface for the network - the standard and unified network interface for industrial robot applications. In: Proceedings of the 41st SICE annual conference, vol. 2. SICE; 2002. https://doi.org/10.1109/SICE.2002.1195288.
146. Mizukawa M, Sakakibara S, Otera N. Implementation and applications of open data network interface "ORiN". In: SICE 2004 annual conference, vol. 2; 2004. p. 1340–3.
147. Muragaki Y, Okamoto J, Saito T, et al. STMO-06 smart cyber operating theater realized by Internet of Things - results of clinical study for 56 cases. Neuro-Oncol Adv. 2019;1:ii19. https://doi.org/10.1093/noajnl/vdz039.086.

Surgeon-Supporting Robots

Tetsuya Goto

1 Introduction

Microscopic and/or endoscopic procedures in neurosurgery are now well established. Sufficient neurosurgical knowledge and surgical skill are indispensable for the success of a difficult surgery. However, to maintain fine and precise maneuvers throughout the surgery is challenging because the surgeon is a human, not a robot. The surgeon's mental and physical condition must affect the results. When the surgeon becomes exhausted, concentration is decreased and mistakes can happen. A surgeon's muscles and joints cannot sustain their positions at the same point over a long time. The attempt leads to increased physiological tremors and perturbs fine movements.

Many types of surgical robots have been developed to perform surgical maneuvers in place of the surgeon's direct actions [1–3]. Robotics researchers believe that the robot can perform more precise procedures than the surgeon; indeed, robots can even perform procedures impossible for surgeons. Robotics-assisted surgery can be used to perform difficult and complex procedures by conventional methods. On the other hand, we recognize that a well-experienced craftsman can make highly exquisite and precise procedures with better than industrial accuracy. Neurosurgeons explain that neurosurgery is an "art" not a "science." Our ultimate goal is not to develop surgical robots but to achieve better surgical results and outcomes using robotics technology.

T. Goto (✉)
Department of Neurosurgery, St. Marianna University School of Medicine,
Kawasaki, Kanagawa, Japan
e-mail: tegotou@marianna-u.ac.jp

© The Author(s), under exclusive license to Springer Nature
Switzerland AG 2022
M. M. Al-Salihi et al. (eds.), *Introduction to Robotics in Minimally Invasive
Neurosurgery*, https://doi.org/10.1007/978-3-030-90862-1_8

In this chapter, two kinds of commercially available robots for supporting surgeons are introduced. Although they never perform surgical procedures by themselves, they maximize the surgeon's ability to achieve precise technique, thus producing flawless procedures.

2   Surgeon's Arm Supporting Robot: iArmS

2.1   Motivation

We have physiological tremor in our hands and fingers, and this develops when the surgeon stretches out the arms and muscle tension in the arm strengthens [4, 5]. The tremor can be reduced by touching a point or reducing the muscle tension. Continuous precise motions of surgical instruments are required in microneurosurgery. Precise movements can be achieved with adequate stabilization of the surgeon's arm in the appropriate position [6, 7]. To achieve adequate stabilization it is important that the surgeon's arm, hand, or fingers be fixed on the craniotomy edge, the head fixation frame, and/or the surgeon's arm be fixed on the armrest of the chair [8–10]. There are many types of armrests, which can be part of the chair or independent of it. A freely movable armrest (FMA) can change its position according to the surgeon's requirements. The smart arm®, one type of FMA, has been commercially available for two decades [11]. The armrest of the smart arm can be moved when the air compression brake in each joint is released by pressing the button manually. The use of the FMA reduces tremor when fine microsurgical movements are performed and thus provides good surgical results.

Despite its advantages for procedural precision, FMA-assisted surgery has not been widely adopted. The optimal position of the surgeon's arm changes frequently. Adjustment of the armrest to the optimal position during the operation can, therefore, be difficult. If the armrest automatically moves and holds the surgeon's arm while the procedure is being performed, that will meet the surgeon's requirements. To achieve this, the iArmS®: auto-adjusting freely movable armrest has been developed [6, 12].

2.2   Materials

The iArmS consists of an arm holder, a robot arm, and a base (Fig. 1) [12–14]. The arm holder has a curved shape and the surgeon puts their forearm on it (Figs. 2 and 3). A force sensor is set between the arm holder and the robot arm.

The robot arm has five degrees of freedom. No electric motors are used in it. Each joint has electric brakes and encoders. The base, which has four moveable wheels, can stand independently. iArmS has three working states: "Free," "Fix," and "Wait." In the "Free" state, the electric brakes are released and the robot arm is moved upwards by the counterweight of each joint so the arm holder pushes the surgeon's arm from below.

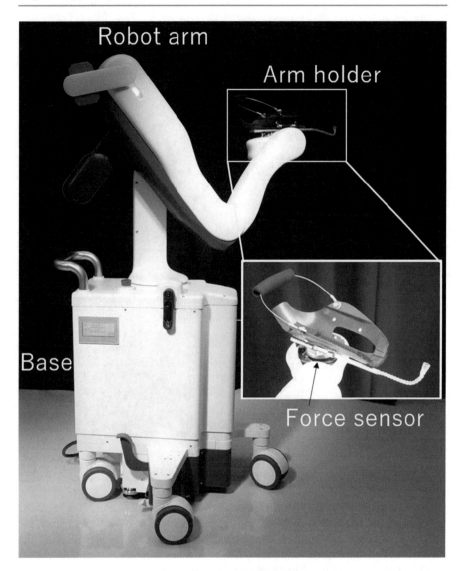

Fig. 1 This figure shows the lateral view of iArmS. The iArmS consists of an arm holder, a robot arm, and a base. A force sensor is placed between the arm holder and the robot arm. It senses the surgeon's movement, and the robot arm is controlled by the information from it. Each shaft of the robot arm is 30 cm long. The total weight of iArmS is 100 kg; it is heavy in order to prevent it from falling

The friction between the surgeon's arm and the arm holder moves iArmS so it follows. In the "Fix" state, the arm holder maintains the position by locking the electric brakes and supports the surgeon's arm weight. When the surgeon's arm moves away from the arm holder, for example, to change surgical instruments or move the operating microscope, it enters the "Wait" state. The arm holder maintains

Fig. 2 This figure shows
the iArmS robot with the
surgeon in a sitting
position. The iArmS is
connected to the surgical
chair and moves with it

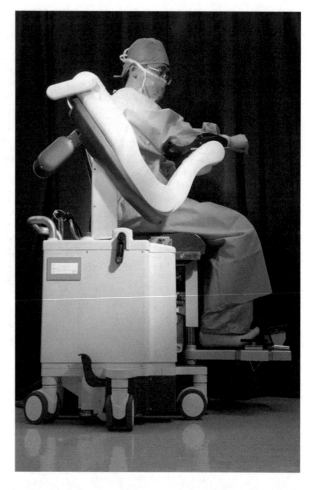

its position by locking the electric brakes. When there is no surgeon's arm on the arm holder and the unit is in "Free" mode, the arm holder moves away from the patient. Each state is converted automatically by analyzing the signals from the force sensor and the encoders in each joint.

The iArmS was produced by DENSO Corporation (Kariya, Japan) in 2016. Now, all rights have been transferred to TOHO engineering corporation (Nagoya, Japan). To date, it has been commercially available only in Japan.

2.3 Users' Evaluation

2.3.1 Maneuverability

Many surgeons recognize that the iArmS reduces the hand tremor during micro-neurosurgery (Fig. 4) [12, 15]. The conventional finger-placing technique used by neurosurgeons to reduce hand tremors is effective. In previous basic experiments it

Fig. 3 This figure shows the frontal view of the iArmS robot with the surgeon in standing position. The height of the robot arm can be adjusted by the base

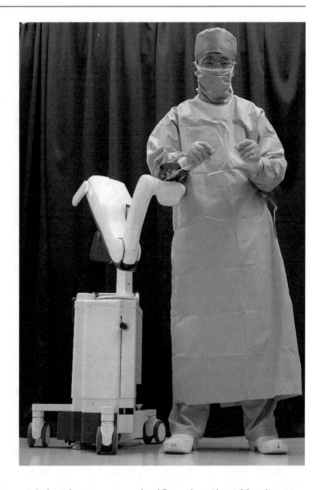

was confirmed that the surgeon's hand tremor was significantly reduced by the arm-rest in the appropriate position [6, 7]. However, under some conditions it cannot always be implemented. In such a situation, iArmS might still be a useful tool. The surgeon who noticed hand tremors without iArmS felt an improvement in tremor when iArmS was used. This result means that the surgeon who has hand tremors in the usual situation can feel a decrease of such tremors when iArmS is used. However, the degree of hand tremor differs among surgeons and situations. Some surgeons, who think they can stabilize their own rising and floating hands without support, might not need to use iArmS [15].

The surgical procedure can be easily accomplished using iArmS [15]. This can be achieved not only by the reduction of hand tremors but also by the wider approach to selection of instruments. The surgical instrument insertion angle is determined by the maneuverability of the instrument by the surgeon's hand stabilization and anatomical correctness. Using iArmS, the surgeon's arm can be supported at the appropriate position. The surgeon can select the instrument insertion angle depending on the determinants of anatomical correctness because their arm can be used without

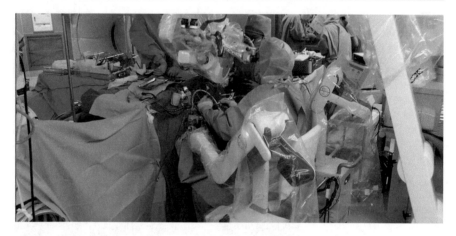

Fig. 4 This figure shows an intraoperative situation during microscopic neurosurgery. The surgeon sits on the surgical chair and two sets of iArmS robots are connected to it. Both arms of the surgeon are placed on the iArmS

tremor or fatigue. iArmS is particularly useful for long shaft instruments such as clip appliers.

Another possibility for using iArmS in neurosurgery is in endoscopic surgery (Fig. 5). The endoscope is held by the surgeon's hand or holding device. The iArmS supports the surgeon's arm holding the endoscope [13]. Stabilization of the surgeon's hand and alleviation of fatigue can facilitate stable and accurate surgery. A scope holder that fixes the endoscope also prevents shaking of the video images. While using a scope holder, the surgeon must stop the surgical procedure while the endoscope is moved to a suitable position [16–18]. Endoscopic neurosurgeons observe the depth of the operative field via two-dimensional video images using "dynamic stereo vision" by allowing the scope to move back and forth slightly. iArmS® both stabilizes the surgeon's hand and provides excellent operability during endoscopic transsphenoidal surgery. Another merit of using iArmS in endoscopic surgery is the prolongation of endoscope lens-wiping intervals and preservation of clear endoscopic vision [17]. Endoscopic surgery is completely dependent on endoscopic images; therefore, the field of view is easily lost if the lens is fouled by the adhesion of fluids [19, 20]. This advantage is also achieved by the stability of the surgeon's hand.

2.3.2 Fatigue

There are multiple reasons for a surgeon's fatigue, not only the performance of a highly complex procedure but also blood loss during the operation, or the operation time (as is known, many neurosurgical operations take very long hours), or communication with the staff. Motivation against surgery can also affect fatigue.

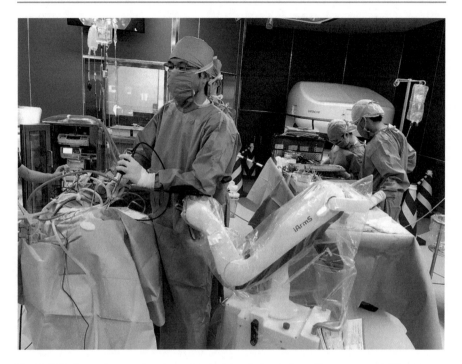

Fig. 5 This figure shows an intraoperative situation during endoscopic neurosurgery. The surgeon is standing beside one iArmS robot. The left hand, which holds the rigid endoscope, is supported by the iArmS. In intraoperative settings, a sterile drape covers the robot arm and the base of the iArmS. The arm holder is reused and sterilized independently to maintain sufficient friction between the surgeon's arm and arm holder

The iArmS can reduce the surgeon's fatigue by supporting the surgeon's arm, thus reducing shoulder and arm tightness. Especially in endoscopic surgery, the surgeon's fatigue can be due to holding the heavy endoscope and concentrating on it. The scope holder can reduce surgeon's fatigue, but surgical maneuverability is decreased. Fatigue can also increase in some surgeons who use iArmS [15]. Although iArmS works automatically, the surgeon must pay attention to it. Fatigue can develop because controlling iArmS is difficult or troublesome. Additional practice in the use of iArmS could help to reduce the surgeon's fatigue.

2.3.3 Demerits
The demerits of iArmS are that the robot is space-occupying and its cost is high, which makes operations using it more expensive. Many surgical tools such as the operative microscope, navigation systems, drilling system, and coagulation system must be set near the surgeon. The base of iArmS is large and heavy enough to prevent the system from falling over, which makes this robot space-occupying and restricts the room for surgeons to move in the theater.

3 Archelis: Surgical Knee Rest

3.1 Motivation

The operative field is static; it can never move, but the visual angle by microscope or endoscope and manipulation angle must be changed frequently. This obliges the surgeon to remain standing in order to be able to move around the operating theater as soon as possible. This obligatory standing posture throughout a long-time operation causes musculoskeletal fatigue and stress [21, 22], intensified by the physical burden on surgeons [23–25]. This can make the surgeon aware throughout the procedure of the difficulty in completing the delicate manipulations required. Using a round chair with a caster and height adjuster cannot meet our requirements, and there are many other disadvantages such as: the chair never follows the surgeon when they stand up; it is a space-occupying structure inside the theater that becomes completely useless when the surgeon decides to move; action is needed to adjust its vertical height, which is time-consuming; and the surgeon must pay attention to the position of the seat while sitting on it. A body and foot supporting device is needed to support the surgeon in the appropriate position during precise procedures. Archelis follows the surgeon without requiring attention, not only in the horizontal plane but also vertically [26–28].

3.2 Materials

The Archelis is a passive exoskeleton device developed by Nitto Co., Ltd. (Yokoyama, Japan) and produced by Olympus Medical Science Sales Co., Ltd. (Tokyo, Japan) and Zimmer Biomet G.K. (Tokyo, Japan). The name "Archelis" is derived from the swiftest-footed hero Achilles in Greek mythology. In Japanese words, "a-r-che-l-is" can be called "a-ru-ke-ru=i-su," which means "walkable chair."

The exoskeleton, literally the external skeleton of insects, is one of the keywords for understanding the robot. Many animals including fish, birds, mammals, and human beings have endoskeletons, the opposite of exoskeletons. The armor that protects the human's body recalls the ancient exoskeleton. There is no way to support extreme movements in humans other than by covering the body surface. There are two kinds of exoskeleton robots, powered and passive. The powered exoskeleton, known as power armor, powered armor, or powered suit, is a wearable mobile machine powered by an electric motor, springs, or damper. The powered exoskeleton senses the user's motion and sends signals to the motors to move the joints of the exoskeleton. It allows for the user's movement with increased strength and endurance. Basic movements of human beings—walking and climbing with a heavy burden, lifting and holding heavy items—can be assisted by a powered exoskeleton.

The exoskeleton technology originally focused on military [29] and rehabilitation applications [30, 31]. A passive exoskeleton has no power assistance. Similar to a powered exoskeleton, it gives mechanical benefits to the user. It is being used increasingly in the automotive industry in order to reduce worker injuries and errors due to fatigue [32, 33].

The Archelis supports the surgeon's lower limb in maintaining a near-standing posture by being worn on the lower half of the body. It consists of an aluminum plate and plastic cover in the hard part. The total weight is approximately 3.2 kg per extremity (Fig. 6). The hard part is fastened by Velcro to the surgeon's femur and lower thigh [34]. The knee part has a joint that can be locked or unlocked.

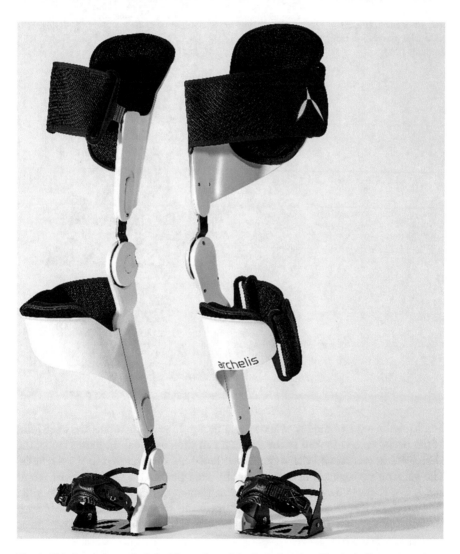

Fig. 6 This figure shows the left oblique view of the Archelis robot. The Archelis consists of two independent right and left parts. Its total weight is approximately 3.2 kg per extremity. The whitish hard part is fastened with Velcro to the surgeon's leg and lower back. (Image used with permission from Archelis Inc.)

Fig. 7 This figure shows
the Archelis worn by a
standing surgeon. The
whitish hard part is
fastened to the surgeon's
leg and lower back by two
sets of black Velcro. The
surgeon is made to feel as
though in a sitting position
by the support on the leg
and lower back. (Image
used with permission from
Archelis Inc.)

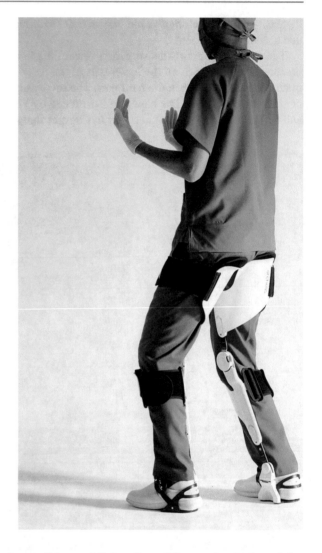

The Archelis has two modes: walking and fixing. In walking mode, the knee joint
of the Archelis is unlocked so the surgeon can walk as usual. In fixing mode, the
knee joint is locked and the surgeon can leave his own burden to the Archelis.
The surgeon's knees are held in a slightly bent position. The support of femur
and lower thigh makes the surgeon feel as though sitting (Fig. 7). The surgeon
puts on the Archelis while dressing in operating clothes and takes it off after
leaving the operating room (Fig. 8). Before skin scrubbing, the Archelis is
adjusted to fixing mode.

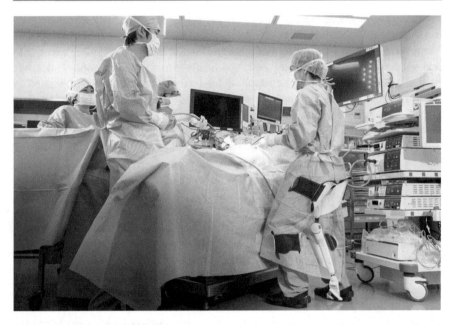

Fig. 8 This figure shows the adaptation of the Archelis robot in intraoperative settings. (Image used with permission from Archelis Inc.)

3.3 Users' Evaluation

In the preliminary report, the surgeons felt relaxed during and after surgery. The Archelis decreased the surgeons' back muscle contractions and improved their work environment, although they felt slight difficulty in walking simultaneously. All surgeons would recommend the Archelis to their colleagues for use during operations [34].

4 Discussion

The industry field is similar to the surgical field in many ways such as considering the applications of robotics technology. Industrial products are equivalent to surgical results; an industrial worker is equivalent to a surgeon; the industrial factory is an operating room. Just as many types of industrial devices work in the factory, many surgical devices are necessary in the operating room. An industrial product is the result of manufacturing processes. Human factors participate strongly in the quality of the products thanks to the capacity for manipulation, dexterity, flexibility, problem-solving, and intelligence. However, they never make a product alone. They need well-established tools, precise machining apparatus, an appropriate work environment and a management body in the factory.

The surgeon needs similar factors in the operating room. All of the surgical devices in the operating room can be regarded as a surgeon-supporting system. Many such devices—operating table, surgical chair, head frame system, and armrest—touch the surgeon's body, feet, and hands directly. Microscope, endoscope holder, and many switches for controlling medical devices are directly operated by the surgeon. Adapting ergonomics design to these devices has the potential to increase the surgeon's manipulative ability. When robotics technology adopts these devices, we can define them as surgeon-supporting robots.

The difference between industry workers and surgeons is protection against fatigue. In industry, the relationship between productivity and human labor has been researched extensively [35–37]. The main approach to maintaining high productivity is appropriate distributions of workload. Most of the literature deals with balancing the assembly line process, distributing the assembly work among the workstations and reducing the total workload [36]. In contrast, the surgeon cannot take a rest during surgery. It is remarkable that much of the literature reveals that surgeons' fatigue does not correlate with surgical outcomes [38, 39]. These conclusions followed investigations into the relationship between surgical outcome and the surgeon's workload or resting time. The quality of industrial products can be decreased by a worker's lack of incentive and carelessness, which is caused by accumulative fatigue. Surgeons strongly believe that such fatigue cannot happen to them during surgery.

Assembly task assignments and ergonomic evaluations are often conducted separately [40, 41]. Extended repetitions of movements in manual tasks can lead to work-related musculoskeletal disorders. With specific regard to the risk of work-related musculoskeletal disorders, the Occupational Repetitive Actions method is widely acknowledged [42]. This method, standardized by ISO (ISO 11228-3 technical standard) and by CEN (EN 1005-5), can be used to estimate the risk for workers employed in highly repetitive manual tasks. Although surgeons hesitate to regard their surgical outcome as being poor because of fatigue, this type of fatigue must also occur among them. We should recognize the effects of fatigue on surgical outcomes and make efforts to reduce musculoskeletal aches during operations.

5   Conclusion

The surgeon-supporting robots never perform a surgical procedure. They only assist the surgeons, as with armrests or chairs. It is therefore difficult to evaluate their effect on surgical outcome. There is less motivation to purchase those surgeon-supporting devices in hospitals than other more important devices, which are "indispensable." Although a surgeon-supporting device can improve the quality of surgery, the need for them differs among surgeons because of their differences in style. These devices should be used only by those who want to use them.

References

1. Hongo K, Kobayashi S, Kakizawa Y, Koyama J, Goto T, Okudera H, Kan K, Fujie MG, Iseki H, Takakura K. NeuRobot: telecontrolled micromanipulator system for minimally invasive microneurosurgery-preliminary results. Neurosurgery. 2002;51(4):985–8. discussion 988.
2. Marcus HJ, Hughes-Hallett A, Cundy TP, Yang GZ, Darzi A, Nandi D. da Vinci robot-assisted keyhole neurosurgery: a cadaver study on feasibility and safety. Neurosurg Rev. 2015;38:367–71.
3. Sutherland GR, Wolfsberger S, Lama S, Zarei-nia K. The evolution of neuroArm. Neurosurgery. 2013 Jan;72(Suppl 1):27–32.
4. Deuschl G, Bain P, Brin M. Ad hoc scientific committee: consensus statement of the movement disorder society on tremor. Mov Disord. 1998;13(Suppl 3):2–23.
5. Elble RJ, Randall JE. Motor-unit activity responsible for 8- to 12-Hz component of human physiological finger tremor. J Neurophysiol. 1976;39:370–83.
6. Yako T, Goto T, Hongo K. Usefulness and limitation of a freely movable armrest in microneurosurgery. Int J Neurol Neurosurg. 2009;1:185–90.
7. Hara Y, Goto T, Okamoto J, Okuda H, Iseki H, Hongo K. An armrest is effective for reducing hand tremble in neurosurgeons. Neurol Med Chir (Tokyo). 2015;55(4):311–6.
8. Klein F. Möller UNIVERSAL operation unit. Neurosurg Rev. 1984;7:99–102.
9. Gilsbach JM, Lutze T, Seeger W. Combined retractor and hand-rest system for microneurosurgery. Neurosurg Rev. 1984;7:85–7.
10. Kobayashi S, Sugita K, Matsuo K. An improved neurosurgical systems: new operating table, chair, microscope and other instrumentation. Neurosurg Rev. 1984;7:75–80.
11. Ohta T, Kuroiwa T. Freely movable armrest for microneurosurgery: technical note. Neurosurgery. 2001;46:1259–61.
12. Goto T, Hongo K, Yako T, Hara Y, Okamoto J, Toyoda K, Fujie MG, Iseki H. The concept and feasibility of EXPERT: intelligent armrest using robotics technology. Neurosurgery. 2013;72(Suppl 1):A39–42.
13. Ogiwara T, Goto T, Nagm A, Hongo K. Endoscopic endonasal transsphenoidal surgery using the iArmS operation support robot: initial experience in 43 patients. Neurosurg Focus. 2017;42:E10.
14. Okuda H, Okamoto J, Takumi Y, Kakehata S, Muragaki Y. The iArmS robotic armrest prolongs endoscope lens-wiping intervals in endoscopic sinus surgery. Surg Innov. 2020;27:515–22.
15. Goto T, Hongo K, Ogiwara T, Nagm A, Okamoto J, Muragaki Y, Lawton M, McDermott M, Berger M. Intelligent surgeon's arm supporting system iArmS in microscopic neurosurgery utilizing robotic technology. World Neurosurg. 2018; pii: S1878-8750(18)31717-0.
16. Morita A, Okada Y, Kitano M, Hori T, Taneda M, Kirino T. Development of hybrid integrated endoscope-holder system for endoscopic microneurosurgery. Neurosurgery. 2004;55:926–32.
17. Eskandari R, Amini A, Yonemura K, Couldwell W. The use of the Olympus EndoArm for spinal and skull-based transsphenoidal neurosurgery. Minim Invasive Neurosurg. 2008;51:370–2.
18. Mamelak AN, Carmichael J, Bonert VH, Cooper O, Melmed S. Single-surgeon fully endoscopic endonasal transsphenoidal surgery: outcomes in three-hundred consecutive cases. Pituitary. 2013;16:393–401.
19. Cassera MA, Goers TA, Spaun GO, Swanström LL. Efficacy of using a novel endoscopic lens cleaning device: a prospective randomized controlled trial. Surg Innov. 2011;18:150–5.
20. Schoofs J, Gossot D. A neglected but frustrating ergonomic issue: the thoracoscopic trocar. Minim Invasive Ther Allied Technol. 2004;13:133–7.
21. Vijendren A, Yung M, Sanchez J. The ill surgeon: a review of common work-related health problems amongst UK surgeons. Langenbeck's Arch Surg. 2014;399(8):967–79.
22. Steinhilber B, Hoffmann S, Karlovic K, et al. Development of an arm support system to improve ergonomics in laparoscopic surgery: study design and provisional results. Surg Endosc. 2015;29(9):2851–8.

23. Nguyen NT, Ho HS, Smith WD, et al. An ergonomic evaluation of surgeons' axial skeletal and upper extremity movements during laparoscopic and open surgery. Am J Surg. 2001;182(6):720–4.
24. Alleblas CCJ, Velthuis S, Nieboer TE, Sietses C, Stegeman DF. The physical workload of surgeons: a comparison of SILS and conventional laparoscopy. Surg Innov. 2015;22(4):376–81.
25. Miller K, Benden M, Pickens A, Shipp E, Zheng Q. Ergonomics principles associated with laparoscopic surgeon injury/illness. Hum Factors. 2012;54(6):1087–92.
26. Emam TA, Hanna G, Cuschieri A. Ergonomic principles of task alignment, visual display, and direction of execution of laparoscopic bowel suturing. Surg Endosc. 2002;16(2):267–71.
27. van Det MJ, Meijerink WJHJ, Hoff C, Totté ER, Pierie JPEN. Optimal ergonomics for laparoscopic surgery in minimally invasive surgery suites: a review and guidelines. Surg Endosc. 2009;23(6):1279–85.
28. Iqbal MH, Aydin A, Brunckhorst O, Dasgupta P, Ahmed K. A review of wearable technology in medicine. J R Soc Med. 2016;109(10):372–80.
29. Zoss AB, Kazerooni H, Chu A. Biomechanical design of the Berkeley lower extremity exoskeleton (BLEEX). IEEE/ASME Trans Mechatr. 2006;11:128–38.
30. Kawamoto H, Sankai Y. Power assist system HAL-3 for gait disorder person. In: Miesenberger K, Klaus J, Zagler W, editors. Computers helping people with special needs. ICCHP 2002. Lecture notes in computer science, vol. 2398. Berlin, Heidelberg: Springer; 2002. p. 196–203.
31. Cruciger O, Schildhauer TA, Meindl RC, et al. Impact of locomotion training with a neurologic controlled hybrid assistive limb (HAL) exoskeleton on neuropathic pain and health related quality of life (HRQoL) in chronic SCI: a case study. Disabil Rehabil Assist Technol. 2014;11(6):1–6.
32. Spadaa S, Ghibaudoa L, Gilottaa S. Laura Gastaldib and Maria pia Cavatorta investigation into the applicability of a passive upper-limb exoskeleton in automotive industry. Proced Manufactur. 2017;11:1255–62.
33. Theurel J, Desbrosses K, Roux T, Savescu A. Physiological consequences of using an upper limb exoskeleton during manual handling tasks. Appl Ergon. 2018;67:211–7.
34. Kawahira H, Nakamura R, Shimomura Y, Oshiro T, Okazumi S, Lefor AK. A wearable lower extremity support for laparoscopic surgeons: a pilot study. Asian J Endosc Surg. 2021;14:144–8.
35. Janaro RE, Bechtold SE. A study of the reduction of fatigue impact on productivity through optimal rest break scheduling. Hum Factors. 1985;27:459–66.
36. Battaia O, Dolgui A. A taxonomy of line balancing problems and their solution ap proaches. Int J Product Econ. 2013;142:259–77.
37. Van den Bergh J, Belien J, De Bruecker P, Demeulemeester E, De Boeck L. Personnel scheduling: a literature review. Eur J Oper Res. 2013;226:367–85.
38. Koda N, Oshima Y, Koda K, Shimada H. Surgeon fatigue does not affect surgical outcomes: a systematic review and meta-analysis. Surg Today. 2020;13 https://doi.org/10.1007/s00595-020-02138-9.
39. Butler KA, Kapetanakis VE, Smith BE, Sanjak M, Verheijde JL, Chang YH, Magtibay PM, Magrina JF. Surgeon fatigue and postural stability: is robotic better than laparoscopic surgery? J Laparoendosc Adv Surg Tech A. 2013;23(4):343–6.
40. Choi G. A goal programming mixed-model line balancing for processing time and physical workload. Comput Indust Eng. 2009;57:395–400.
41. Otto A, Scholl A. Incorporating ergonomic risks into assembly line balancing. Eur J Oper Res. 2011;212:277–85.
42. Colombini D, Occhipinti E, Grieco A. Risk assessment and management of repetitive movements and exertions of upper limbs. Oxford: Elsevier; 2002. ISBN: 9780080440804

Augmented and Virtual Reality Training Simulators for Robotic Neurosurgery

Sandrine de Ribaupierre and Roy Eagleson

1   Introduction

There has been a rapid increase in the use of robotic surgery across a number of disciplines during the past quarter century. Some robotic systems were adopted early in specific neurosurgical categories; however, more general adoption across a broad range of neurosurgery disciplines has been slower [1]. Neurosurgical robots are discussed in other chapters of this book, so this chapter will highlight specific examples of systems in which augmented reality (AR) or virtual reality (VR) is used for training.

Before discussing the use of AR and VR, we can review some previous cases in which robotic arms in cranial neurosurgery were used in the 1990s, followed by commercial models such as the Neuromate® (Renishaw, UK), which was approved in 1999 by the FDA, and the ROSA® BRAIN robot (Medtch/Zimmer Biomet, France). These varieties of robotic arm systems enable surgeons to plan their trajectory based on imaging, and then follow that plan once it is registered. They facilitate stereotactic surgeries with or without frames.

Similar systems have been used in spine surgery, following the development of a PUMA-based surgical robot in 1992, allow the surgeon to specify a precise trajectory for drilling in spine fixation [2]. Another example is the SpineAssist (Mazor Robotics Ltd., Caesarea, Israel) with many subsequent extensions (Renaissance, Mazor X).

S. de Ribaupierre (✉)
Department of Clinical Neurological Sciences, Schulich School of Medicine and Dentistry, and Brain and Mind Institute, University of Western Ontario, London, ON, Canada
e-mail: sderibau@uwo.ca

R. Eagleson
Electrical and Computer Engineering, and Brain and Mind Institute, University of Western Ontario, London, ON, Canada
e-mail: eagleson@uwo.ca

© The Author(s), under exclusive license to Springer Nature
Switzerland AG 2022
M. M. Al-Salihi et al. (eds.), *Introduction to Robotics in Minimally Invasive Neurosurgery*, https://doi.org/10.1007/978-3-030-90862-1_9

We can focus on a different category, of surgical procedures, making use of tele-operated robotic systems, such as the da Vinci Surgical System®, developed by Intuitive Surgical (Sunnyvale, USA) and used for laparoscopic surgery since 2000. More recently, this system has been used for anterior approaches in spinal surgery such as anterior lumbar interbody fusions (ALIF), transoral odontoidectomies or resection of thoracolumbar neurofibromas. Another example is the NeuroArm®, developed in Calgary [3]; the first case was performed in 2008. Tele-robotic systems enable the surgeon to operate from a different room and can also be used when the patient is in a CT or MRI bore. Force sensors are built into the system and the manipulandum position data are filtered to reduce hand tremor. There are also newer, smaller robots that are slowly being integrated in neurosurgical practice. For example, for transsphenoidal surgery, a Japanese team has developed the Smart Arm, a versatile arm for constrained spaces, able, for example, to perform dural suturing [4].

One can also think of robot-guided microscopes or exoscopes (Synaptive, Modus V) where the focus, field of view, and lighting can be adjusted automatically. Other robotic arms enable the surgeon to retract an area or to rest their arms while working in order to reduce tremor.

All these systems present different Use Cases for augmented reality (AR)/virtual reality (VR) training; but in each of them, the surgeon needs to be trained to use the system in order to be fully aware of the mapping from the OR contextual workspace, to the inner workspace, and to be able to control the location and trajectory of the surgical tool in relation to the inner surgical workspace. This forms the overarching motivation for considering AR and VR simulators for Surgical Training.

2 Design of Augmented and Virtual Reality Simulators for Surgical Training

Augmented reality (AR) involves a display of supplementary graphic information superimposed on the display of a real surface or a phantom. For example, one can project a tumor and blood vessels on to a plastic skull or a 3D printed PVC brain phantom; and in the workspace, real instruments can be used [5]. In contrast, virtual reality (VR) is a totally immersive environment in which everything is simulated and visualized through a computer graphic, including the tools used for surgery [6]. Mixed reality (MR) is the display of computer-generated images on a real surface, as in AR, but the real-world objects are "spatially aware and responsive," allowing full interaction with the projected images.

The overarching premise for developing AR- and VR-based surgical training system comes not only from the broad interest seen in the literature for developing a range of projects examining the use of such systems. More importantly, we can suggest why this interest has developed by considering the opportunity that such systems provide for gathering objective metrics to evaluate them.

For any surgical procedure, the formal "complexity" is reflected in the hierarchical representation of that procedure. It comprises nested tasks and subtasks, the lowest level having a base defined in terms of visual-motor primitives, which are either movements through space or interactions between tool and tissue [7]. These human-directed motor outputs are guided by visual information, which allows the free-space movements to be guided in 3D or enables the interaction of the surgical tools with the patient's body to be judged (sometimes in conjunction with haptic feedback).

Accordingly, at the lowest visual-motor level of abstraction, AR and VR presentations of simulated tool interactions with patient anatomical models can be used to train up the psychomotor skills of the resident or surgeon. Currently, VR seems more suitable for this purpose than AR, which seems to bring increased challenges with depth perception in surgical skills learning [8–11]. Broadly speaking, pure AR systems are notorious for difficulties in generating scenes which mix 'real' and 'graphical' content in a way that does not cause conflicting visual depth cues, giving them poor usabililty for interactive manipulation of items seen in the workspace.

Furthermore, when implementing systems for controlling visual/motor tasks at this low level of surgical interaction, where all aspects of the procedure are decomposed into visual-motor free-space movements or tool-body interactions–we are able to specify formal metrics for performance that are expressed in terms of either the speed and accuracy of the movement phases or the decision-theoretical times and error rates for the interactions that require judgment (decisions about the adequacy of the tool-tissue interaction).

As we move up the visual-motor abstraction hierarchy to consider the different categories of surgical procedure, we will continue our review of the literature in terms of three different categories of robots available for surgery:

1. a supervisory controlled system in which the robot performs actions based on a surgical plan that is made using imaging;
2. a tele-surgery system using a haptic system interface in real time where the robot replicates the surgeon's movement from the interface;
3. a shared control system where the surgeon has full control, and the robot assists, symbiotically, in hand manipulation of the instrument.

Each category has specific training requirements, which can all be taught and assessed using a VR system.

In the first category of the controlled arm, where a plan is devised by the surgeon using imaging and then executed by the robot, which will guide the surgeon to the trajectory, education is about ensuring that the surgeon can form an overarching surgical plan, verify the accuracy of the system, and recognize any issues during mobilization of the arm. Some of the skills are the same as those involved in using a neuronavigation system, and therefore most neurosurgeons become acquainted with them during residency training. Some local research groups might be evaluating VR systems for training these skills, but currently there are no widely available or commercial systems. Extension of accuracy methods for AR surgical navigation [12] could be used to train virtually with robotic arms. In VR, or a mixture of VR and AR/MR, the complete surgery can be implemented as a module with different

Flowchart of insertion of SEEG electrodes

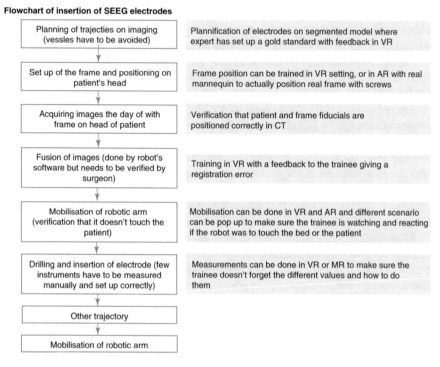

| Planning of trajecties on imaging (vessles have to be avoided) | Plannification of electrodes on segmented model where expert has set up a gold standard with feedback in VR |

| Set up of the frame and positioning on patient's head | Frame position can be trained in VR setting, or in AR with real mannequin to actually position real frame with screws |

| Acquiring images the day of with frame on head of patient | Verification that patient and frame fiducials are positioned correctly in CT |

| Fusion of images (done by robot's software but needs to be verified by surgeon) | Training in VR with a feedback to the trainee giving a registration error |

| Mobilisation of robotic arm (verification that it doesn't touch the patient) | Mobilisation can be done in VR and AR and different scenario can be pop up to make sure the trainee is watching and reacting if the robot was to touch the bed or the patient |

| Drilling and insertion of electrode (few instruments have to be measured manually and set up correctly) | Measurements can be done in VR or MR to make sure the trainee doesn't forget the different values and how to do them |

Other trajectory

Mobilisation of robotic arm

Fig. 1 Example of a flowchart for SEEG electrode insertion using a robot. On the left, the different steps. On the right, the steps that could be implemented in a VR simulation

steps to be followed. The trainee receives feedback throughout and not only learns the multiple steps but can also assess the accuracy of the planning, the fusion, and the trajectory (Fig. 1).

The second category, using haptic devices as an interface and having the robot replicate the movements of the surgeon, necessitates special surgical skills. These systems are typically designed to require a dedicated VR trainer. They include the da Vinci (da Vinci skills simulator "dVSS") [13], the NeuroArm, and the SmartArm (Fig. 2). Typically, haptics-enabled robotic systems involve a steep learning curve: in these master–slave systems, the surgeon learns to manipulate the robot distally through manipulandum as the master and graspers as the slave. The teams that developed these systems quickly understood the needs of a dedicated VR training system in order for the surgeon to learn to perform the movements and control the robot. The trainee starts by performing simple "peg in hole" tasks on the trainer, such as moving pieces around, followed by manipulation of surgical instruments (scissors, forceps, etc.) (Fig. 2). In addition to the dedicated training systems provided by the robotic company, other commercial robotic training systems have emerged (Robotic surgical simulator RoSS™, Mimic dV-TrainerdV-Trainer®, SimSurgery Educational Platform SEP) [14]. Studies show that training on the mimic trainer or da Vinci system does improve some skills using the robot [15].

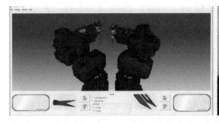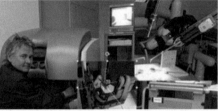

Fig. 2 Examples of VR simulators. On the left, an example of the Neuroarm simulator software; instruments can be selected and changed (here, scissors and scalpel). On the right, a picture of the 3D VR DaVinci simulator

Here, the VR system is focused on learning to manipulate the robot with the graspers or haptic devices, so the simulator can provide direct feedback on the forces used and how the task was achieved (some examples would be: regularity of sutures or knots; completion of dissection of arachnoid threats around a tumor). However, a curriculum can also be developed with increasingly difficult cases, or the addition of unplanned events such as a bleed, or brain shift, or a patient waking up, to teach the trainee how to deal with such challenges (as you would see in the aviation world where pilots have to deal with a defective engine or an unplanned landing).

For the third category, where the robot is a shared system and assists the surgeon by retracting an area or supporting the surgeon's arms to decrease fatigue, specific training is again necessary with the robot, or a VR platform, in order to develop skills for manipulating the robot.

In the case of an exoscope, with a robotic component helping to focus and light the work area, the surgeon performs a procedure while looking at a screen instead of directly into the microscope, as most surgeons have been trained to do. Therefore, training in this skill using an AR or VR system will also decrease the learning curve on patients [16]. Once again, VR and AR will enable a curriculum with increasing difficulties to be designed and to cope with some unplanned events.

All of these training skills could hypothetically be performed on cadavers, animals or 3D printed models, using the real robot. However, this entails logistical issues such as time of training, which should be done after hours when the OR with the robot is available. It also raises the issue of working with cadaveric or animal material in the same space and with the same instruments used for surgery, with a small risk of contamination (prion disease, etc.). Therefore, the design of VR training can be quite advantageous. There can be initial costs linked to the design of the VR simulator, but this can then be made to cost less than the real robot. Accordingly, the costs associated with its use can be decreased. Access to the OR is not required in those cases, and trainees can access the system at any time. Furthermore, there are no cadaveric or 3D model costs.

We have already highlighted the fact that specific curricula can easily be designed and targeted to the skills of the trainee, and cases with increasing difficulties as well as unplanned events can be included. In addition, feedback can be provided to the user in terms of performance, and trainees can track their own performance over time.

VR teaching also has other advantages. For example, using a dual platform as allowed by the da Vinci system, the trainee and the instructor have not only the same view but also the same "hands," and the instructor can take control to show the trainee how to perform a maneuver.

VR systems have an added advantage: they enable session recordings and trajectory logfiles to be gathered, facilitating debriefing or review of the sessions. A specific portion of the surgery can be repeated over again, and the rest of the procedure can be skipped in order to gain time during training so only the critical phases are emphasized. As all individuals differ and have personal surgical skills, the difficulties in a specific surgery could arise at different time points, and VR training allows for that flexibility. In addition, these systems can provide a graded set of difficulty levels, or can introduce anatomical variations, and provide the ability to rehearse directly on the anatomy of the specific patient based on pre-operative scans.

3   Objective Metrics and Evaluation of AR- and VR-Based Surgical Training

While a scoring system on the simulator is easily implemented by developers, it is difficult to judge whether mastery of the surgery on the simulator translates effectively into skills during real surgery performed on a human using a robot [17]. One also has to realize that the metrics provided by the simulator are quite different from the feedback that an expert surgeon would provide when teaching a trainee in the operating room. Keeping that in mind, one needs not only to understand the training requirement of the surgeries performed, and the technique of the robot, in order to design an efficient training system; but also to know the trainee's curriculum and to gamify the training in order for the system to be used [7, 18].

Laparoscopic trainers have been available for years, helping residents to learn simple tasks before proceeding to more complex ones; but until "bootcamp" competitions were introduced, most systems were left dormant in a lab space. Having constructive feedback where the trainees can see their progress, but also eventually be in competition with other trainees, helps them to engage with the practice.

While an expert in robotic surgery might only want to rehearse a specific case, not needing that extra layer of design or curriculum, training residents or even surgeons who have never used the robot needs to start with easy tasks and progress to more difficult ones. A curriculum therefore needs to be built by experts instead of just having single tasks available on the simulator. An expert panel can be used to converge on the skills that should be covered and how they could be taught [19–21]. The panel can also decide the weight given to specific assessment metrics to give a final score to the trainee.

Objective metrics to evaluate the trainee can be based on time needed to finish the case, number of errors (which have to be classified according to their severity and weighted into the score), and completeness of the task, but can also take account of the force used on the graspers, and the final result (such as registration error or the co-registration of two images, amount of tumor left behind, amount of normal brain injured, forces applied on normal brain tissue, etc.). Such scores will inevitably involve some subjectivity as it is difficult to quantify how each error would affect a real patient, but they will help by allowing the trainees to have some metric to compare to others or to themselves and to judge their progress.

Finally, to evaluate the simulator itself and whether it is an efficient teaching tool, one has to consider different facets. While a specific simulator should have been subjected to validity testing to determine whether is an efficient teaching tool, it is typically commercialized before being fully studied.

Multiple studies in other surgical specialties have examined face validity (do the simulator tests seem, according to experts, to test what they are supposed to?) and content validity (is the simulator training a range of low-level skills that are deemed important, and is it useful as a training tool?), using a questionnaire to rate the simulator, experts typically giving a subjective score [22–25], but if the questionnaire is well-designed, it can be used to try to elicit responses from experts such as "how can this system be better integrated into the training curriculum?", and "Why would you feel this is a useful training tool?". Keep in mind that measures of 'where', 'when', and 'which', are best answered using objective metrics of position, time, and classification scores – whereas questions of 'why' and 'how' can never be measured objectively – and so this should be the role played by subjective queryeds and qualitative methodologies. Finally, "Construct validity" is quite often treated as if it was a measure of the difference between experts and novices on the simulator – is often tested by comparing performance across groups, having trainees of different levels and experts using the system [26–28]. In fact, "Construct Validity" really should be reserved for the kind of long-term converging sets of research results which strive to discern whether a "construct" is actually being measured in a way that meaningful inferences can be drawn from its constituent metrics. In our research domain, we propose that the construct that we are all trying to measure is called "Surgical Skill" – and so we need to strive to show, over long-term studies, that our measures of speed, accuracy, and detection/classification scores, are gathered from tasks which are representative of a range, whose 'content validity' is spanning appropriately.

Other studies have looked at criterion validity (does a test correlate with an established standard?). This can then be divided into two types: concurrent and predictive validity. For concurrent validity of the simulators (whether different scoring systems or simulators would rate the skills the same way), the exercise is hard; in contrast to psychological tests for which an established standard has been tested for years, there is no established evaluation procedure for an apprenticeship training system such as surgery. Therefore, some of those studies are based only on questionnaires that are usually written with inbuilt bias and sometimes rated by novices. The tasks used to compare experts and novices are different in most studies, and so are the methods used to assess them. Also, while time for completion might correlate with level of expertise in most tasks, some studies have shown no correlation between simulator and robot for different tasks [29–33]. Only a few studies have considered at whether the metrics provided by the simulator correlate with a subjective assessment by the expert [34, 35]. Even fewer studies have been done for predictive validity (whether a high score on the simulator predicts ability to perform the surgery well) [36–38].

4 Future Directions

In order for a training system to be used at different levels and included in a residency curriculum, it should be developed with a curriculum in mind, and therefore developed in collaboration with program directors or educators in neurosurgery. Different steps should have increasing difficulty levels, but the system should be presented engagingly. While there is no need to enhance the environment with game-like features for the rehearsal of a specific case by an expert surgeon, a VR system will benefit from instilling the competitive edge provided by games if it is to be used for training residents. More studies on the effectiveness of translation of skills acquired on simulators into the operating room are necessary; and any new VR simulator should undergo all validity studies before being integrated into a curriculum or used to qualify surgeons as robotic experts. Our main concern with AR-based training systems is the challenges which, to date, still are preventing usable depth perception in mixed-reality scenes.

As in other disciplines (urology and general surgery are pioneers in this matter), widespread adoption of robotic surgery will necessitate the development of a credentialing system. Such a system was developed in laparoscopic surgery with the Fundamentals of Laparoscopic Surgery (FLS), which is required by the American Board of Surgery [39]. This could be done through the residency program as it is for other surgical skills, through mini-fellowships or through different national bootcamp initiatives.

An important step forward, mostly aimed at expert robotic surgeons, would be the easy integration of patient-specific data in order to train on specific patients and rehearse a difficult case before undertaking the surgery.

5 Conclusion

As described in this chapter, augmented and virtual reality simulators can provide an efficient way to train for robotic surgery. However, before they are used in a credentialing framework, as has already been done with laparoscopy in general surgery and is starting to be done in urology for robotic surgery, there is the need for experts to create a structured, competency-based curriculum specifically designed for robotic neurosurgery. Further development of current simulators, in terms of depth perception within interactive mixed reality workspaces, is needed for that goal to be achieved, in addition to allowing surgeons to train using patient-specific data for surgical planning.

References

1. Stumpo V, Staartjes VE, Klukowska AM, et al. Global adoption of robotic technology into neurosurgical practice and research. Neurosurg Rev. 2020; https://doi.org/10.1007/s10143-020-01445-6.

2. Smith JA, Jivraj J, Wong R, Yang V. 30 years of neurosurgical robots: review and trends for manipulators and associated navigational systems. Ann Biomed Eng. 2016;44(4):836–46.

3. Sutherland GR, Wolfsberger S, Lama S, Zarei-nia K. The evolution of neuroArm. Neurosurgery. 2013;72(Suppl 1):27–32.

4. Marinho MM, Harada K, Morita A, Mitsuishi M. SmartArm: integration and validation of a versatile surgical robotic system for constrained workspaces. Int J Med Robot. 2020;16(2):e2053.

5. Abhari K, Baxter JSH, Chen ECS, et al. Training for planning tumour resection: augmented reality and human factors. IEEE Trans Biomed Eng. 2015;62(6):1466–77.

6. Alaraj A, Lemole MG, Finkle JH, et al. Virtual reality training in neurosurgery: review of current status and future applications. Surg Neurol Int. 2011;2(1):52.

7. Eagleson R, de Ribaupierre S, King S, Stroulia E. Medical education through virtual worlds: the HLTHSIM project. Stud Health Technol Inform. 2011;163:180–4.

8. Ribaupierre S, Eagleson R. Editorial: challenges for the usability of AR and VR for clinical neurosurgical procedures. Healthc Technol Lett. 2017;4(5):151.

9. Eagleson R, de Ribaupierre S. Visual perception and human–computer interaction in surgical augmented and virtual reality environments. In: Mixed and augmented reality in medicine. CRC Press; 2018. p. 83–98.

10. Ghandorh H, Mackenzie J, Eagleson R, de Ribaupierre S. Development of augmented reality training simulator systems for neurosurgery using model-driven software engineering. In: 2017 IEEE 30th Canadian conference on electrical and computer engineering (CCECE). IEEE; 2017.

11. Wright T, Ribaupierre S, Eagleson R. Design and evaluation of an augmented reality simulator using leap motion. Healthc Technol Lett. 2017;4(5):210–5.

12. Burström G, Nachabe R, Persson O, Edström E, ElmiTerander A. Augmented and virtual reality instrument tracking for minimally invasive spine surgery: a feasibility and accuracy study: a feasibility and accuracy study. Spine (Phila Pa 1976). 2019;44(15):1097–104.

13. Walliczek-Dworschak U, Mandapathil M, Förtsch A, et al. Structured training on the da Vinci Skills Simulator leads to improvement in technical performance of robotic novices. Clin Otolaryngol. 2017;42(1):71–80.

14. Julian D, Tanaka A, Mattingly P, Truong M, Perez M, Smith R. A comparative analysis and guide to virtual reality robotic surgical simulators. Int J Med Robot. 2018;14(1):e1874.

15. Lerner MA, Ayalew M, Peine WJ, Sundaram CP. Does training on a virtual reality robotic simulator improve performance on the da Vinci surgical system? J Endourol. 2010;24(3):467–72.

16. Hafez A, Haeren RHL, Dillmann J, Laakso A, Niemelä M, Lehecka M. Comparison of operating microscope and exoscope in a highly challenging experimental setting. World Neurosurg. 2020; https://doi.org/10.1016/j.wneu.2020.12.093.

17. Bric JD, Lumbard DC, Frelich MJ, Gould JC. Current state of virtual reality simulation in robotic surgery training: a review. Surg Endosc. 2016;30(6):2169–78.

18. Ribaupierre S, Kapralos B, Haji FA, Stroulia E, Dubrowski A, Eagleson R. Healthcare training enhancement through virtual reality and serious game. In: Ma M, Jain LC, Anderson P, editors. Virtual, augmented reality and serious games for healthcare. Springer; 2014. p. 6–27.

19. Dell'Oglio P, Turri F, Larcher A, et al. Definition of a structured training curriculum for robot-assisted radical cystectomy with intracorporeal ileal conduit in male patients: a Delphi consensus study led by the ERUS educational board. Eur Urol Focus. 2021; https://doi.org/10.1016/j.euf.2020.12.015.

20. Haji FA, Dubrowski A, Drake J, de Ribaupierre S. Needs assessment for simulation training in neuroendoscopy: a Canadian national survey: clinical article. J Neurosurg. 2013;118(2):250–7.

21. Zaika O, Boulton M, Eagleson R, Ribaupierre S. Understanding aneurysm coiling in practice: a delphi inquiry into expert perception. J Federat Am Scoiet Exper Biol. 2019;33(S1)
22. Gavazzi A, Bahsoun AN, Van Haute W, et al. Face, content and construct validity of a virtual reality simulator for robotic surgery (SEP Robot). Ann R Coll Surg Engl. 2011;93(2):152–6.
23. Lyons C, Goldfarb D, Jones SL, et al. Which skills really matter? Proving face, content, and construct validity for a commercial robotic simulator. Surg Endosc. 2013;27(6):2020–30.
24. Perrenot C, Perez M, Tran N, et al. The virtual reality simulator dV-Trainer(®) is a valid assessment tool for robotic surgical skills. Surg Endosc. 2012;26(9):2587–93.
25. Ramos P, Montez J, Tripp A, Ng CK, Gill IS, Hung AJ. Face, content, construct and concurrent validity of dry laboratory exercises for robotic training using a global assessment tool: dry lab exercises for robotic training using global assessment tool. BJU Int. 2014;113(5):836–42.
26. Connolly M, Seligman J, Kastenmeier A, Goldblatt M, Gould JC. Validation of a virtual reality-based robotic surgical skills curriculum. Surg Endosc. 2014;28(5):1691–4.
27. Hung AJ, Zehnder P, Patil MB, et al. Face, content and construct validity of a novel robotic surgery simulator. J Urol. 2011;186(3):1019–24.
28. Raza SJ, Froghi S, Chowriappa A, et al. Construct validation of the key components of Fundamental Skills of Robotic Surgery (FSRS) curriculum--a multi-institution prospective study. J Surg Educ. 2014;71(3):316–24.
29. Hung AJ, Shah SH, Dalag L, Shin D, Gill IS. Development and validation of a novel robotic procedure specific simulation platform: partial nephrectomy. J Urol. 2015;194(2):520–6.
30. Hertz AM, George EI, Vaccaro CM, Brand TC. Head-to-head comparison of three virtual-reality robotic surgery simulators. JSLS. 2018;22(1):e2017.00081.
31. Lee JY, Mucksavage P, Kerbl DC, Huynh VB, Etafy M, McDougall EM. Validation study of a virtual reality robotic simulator--role as an assessment tool? J Urol. 2012;187(3):998–1002.
32. Foell K, Furse A, Honey RJD, Pace KT, Lee JY. Multidisciplinary validation study of the da Vinci Skills Simulator: educational tool and assessment device. J Robot Surg. 2013;7(4):365–9.
33. Leijte E, de Blaauw I, Rosman C, Botden SMBI. Assessment of validity evidence for the RobotiX robot assisted surgery simulator on advanced suturing tasks. BMC Surg. 2020;20(1):183.
34. Dubin AK, Smith R, Julian D, Tanaka A, Mattingly P. A comparison of robotic simulation performance on basic virtual reality skills: simulator subjective versus objective assessment tools. J Minim Invasive Gynecol. 2017;24(7):1184–9.
35. Dubin AK, Julian D, Tanaka A, Mattingly P, Smith R. A model for predicting the GEARS score from virtual reality surgical simulator metrics. Surg Endosc. 2018;32(8):3576–81.
36. Almarzouq A, Hu J, Noureldin YA, et al. Are basic robotic surgical skills transferable from the simulator to the operating room? A randomized, prospective, educational study. Can Urol Assoc J. 2020;14(12):416–22.
37. Hung AJ, Patil MB, Zehnder P, et al. Concurrent and predictive validation of a novel robotic surgery simulator: a prospective, randomized study. J Urol. 2012;187(2):630–7.
38. Shim JS, Noh TI, Kim JY, et al. Predictive validation of a robotic virtual reality simulator: the Tube 3 module for practicing vesicourethral anastomosis in robot-assisted radical prostatectomy. Urology. 2018;122:32–6.
39. Hafford ML, Van Sickle KR, Willis RE. Ensuring competency: are fundamentals of laparoscopic surgery training and certification necessary for practicing surgeons and operating room personnel? Surg Endosc. 2013;27(1):118–26.

Future Directions of Robotics in Neurosurgery

Sorayouth Chumnanvej

1 Introduction

Humans are improving the world thanks to exceptional intelligence, superiority, and efficiency in solving problems. Improvement in almost all relevant sectors has been remarkable and immensely supportive. Extensive developments in the medical sciences during the last few decades have helped to improve our life expectancy [1, 2] and provided us with superior health care. However, certain human limitations—mental, physiological, psychological, and physical—cannot be overcome with our present abilities. Accuracy, precision, and speed remain the most important aspects of our development and abilities. We have reached a stage where we require improvements beyond our physical and mental capabilities in these three aspects. Hence, numerous supportive and automated devices are being invented and developed to overcome these limitations on our development. The applications of computer machines with established systematic protocols have been automated since the previous century. Different uses of computational automation and robotics have now changed the world and our perception of its development. Robotics, once limited to the realm of imagination or science fiction, has become a reality and a tremendous benefit for humans in applications from heavy construction to precision-guided surgical procedures [3]. The potential of real-time application of robotics is unlimited and could entirely change the world as we see it today. Practical, precise, and cautious robotics applications could have far-reaching effects on human life. It is interesting that robotics has become part of both heavy and rough industrial applications and precisely conducted surgical processes for saving lives.

S. Chumnanvej (✉)
Neurosurgery Division, Surgery Department, Faculty of Medicine Ramathibodi Hospital,
Mahidol University, Bangkok, Thailand
e-mail: sorayouth.chu@mahidol.edu

© The Author(s), under exclusive license to Springer Nature
Switzerland AG 2022
M. M. Al-Salihi et al. (eds.), *Introduction to Robotics in Minimally Invasive
Neurosurgery*, https://doi.org/10.1007/978-3-030-90862-1_10

2 Industrial Robots

The application of robotic systems is increasing because of the ease of operation, reduction of risks, reduced production or task completion time, improved automation, better precision, and capacity to avoid human errors. The development of artificial intelligence and computational learning has helped further in promoting the reliability of robotic tool performances [4]. The new age is industrial 4.0, and an industrial revolution has already occurred to integrate and apply digital information, mechanical information, and electrical and electronic processes for the further benefit of human life. Efficient and high-speed transmission and management of digital information is an important facet of this industrial revolution [5]. Similarly, artificial intelligence has had a major effect on improvements in the healthcare sector in the age of industrial revolution 4.0 [6]. Remarkable improvements in advanced sensor technologies, extended applications of artificial intelligence (AI), development of the internet of robotics things (IoRT), growing usage of cloud robotics, and improvement in the architecture of cognitive and cyber-physical robotics have built novel application platforms of advanced robotics [6]. Apart from these latest developments, the number of robotic applications is growing in various industrial contexts, including manufacturing, human–robot collaborations, and synchronous and cooperative robotic performance.

3 Robots in Surgery

Surgery is considered one of the most important responsibilities requiring pivotal precision, adequate professional training, accuracy, and timely decision-making. There are examples of outstanding surgeries that illustrate the remarkable ability and professional competence of a trained surgeon. However, in certain aspects, human efficiency requires adequate technological support for successful outcomes. The limitation of human vision is one such hindrance for delicate surgical processes. Other roadblocks include a high level of steadiness and other factors that can effectively determine the outcome of a procedure. Along with many extraordinary inventions, robotics has become one effective tool in improving visual capacity, steadiness, and improved precision in operations. Our current reliance on robotics has emerged gradually [7], it has been built on several failed attempts at applications and numerous intricate and complicated developments of sensors and communication technologies. In almost all complicated surgeries nowadays, robotic applications have found important roles and applications. These applications include robotic assistance and support in pediatric urology [8], hip arthroplasty [9], shape sensing and catheter control [10], general urological surgeries [11], complicated cardiological process such as the operation of the mitral annulus [12], and esophagectomy [13]. In complex procedures such as neurovascular surgeries [14], thymectomy [15], and ablation of abnormal neurological tissues [16], robotics has recently been used successfully.

3.1   History of Robotic Surgery

The urge to apply robotic techniques in complex and risky surgical procedures was initiated almost 30 years ago because of the requirement for better accuracy and precision, telepresence, and repetitive task completion in such procedures [17]. The first robot used in the operating theater was PUMA 200 (Westinghouse Electric, Pittsburgh, PA) in 1985. It obtained brain biopsies efficiently [18, 19]. The subsequent evolution of robotic systems helped in developing a "master–slave" human–robot system during the 1990s. Integration of computer-aided design and computer-aided manufacture (CAD-CAM) allowed better robots such as ROBODOC [20] to be developed; this was used extensively for arthroplasty and similar surgeries requiring precise 3D structural information for implantation. Remote controlling and precise instruction feeding became feasible during this development. Several important features of robotic surgery that transcended human abilities then allowed robotics to become a regular part of the operating theater. Such abilities included 3D vision, high-quality image streaming, image display with ease of understanding, physiological tremor filtering, runtime motion capturing and scaling, EndoWrist instruments, and other specialized features developed on the basis of specific requirements. The development and application of Automated Endoscopic System for Optimal Positioning (AESOP) during the 1990s, an effective telesurgical robot approved by the FDA, further raised expectations and the telecontrol of robots during major surgery [21]. No account of the progress of robotic surgery would be complete without mentioning the daVinci® surgical system, a total surgical robotic system that is now being used extensively throughout the world. It has been involved in six million surgeries since the 1990s (Source: Intuitive internal data).

3.2   FDA Evaluation and Regulation of Robotically-Assisted Surgical (RAS/RASD) Devices

The growing role of robotics in different aspects of surgery is inevitable following their successful implementation in improving patient care. However, "with great power comes great responsibilities." Excessive application of the latest robotic technologies could cause unwanted complications and compromise the overall goal of patient benefit and healthcare. Hence, proper regulatory measures need to be developed under strict guidelines, and the implementation and use of robotics in surgery should be monitored. Since the first approved robotic surgery using the AESOP system, the FDA has continuously developed guidelines and regulations for proper application of robotic surgical systems. All types of RAS have been clearly defined by the FDA as potentially containing the following:

1. A control system or console for the surgeon for better visualization and movement of the instruments.
2. Surgical instruments that are controlled by the surgeon from proximity or distance through a computerized system, which can have mechanical arms, camera,
   and similar instruments used for the surgery.
3. All supportive units including hardware and software, endoscope, pumps and
   suction units, electrosurgical units, and light sources.

The FDA has allowed precise applications by trained professionals for various
types of regular surgeries using a robot-assisted system. Specific recommendations
and mandates have been provided for healthcare providers and patients in relation
to RAS/RASD. Healthcare providers have been instructed to report adverse events
due to the use of RAS. However, the growing application of the RAS/RASD system
for cancer patients compelled the FDA to publish additional safety regulations on
February 28, 2019, which restricted the use of these techniques in some common
cancer scenarios including hysterectomy, colectomy, and prostatectomy for patients
having short-term (30 day) follow-ups [22, 23]. In response to growing reports of
injuries due to robot-assisted surgery, the FDA has further improved the reporting
system for authentic, verified information. A Medical Product Safety Network
(MedSun) small sample survey was conducted by the FDA to update the regular
challenges faced by modern surgeons responsible for handling RAS/RASD systems
and for having a broad user viewpoint.

3.3   Surgical Robots and Telemedicine

Telemedicine has become a potential method of treatment in the digital age, benefiting the patient and the physician by saving time and allowing easy access to one-on-
one communication. Telerobotics has become an essential part of telemedicine and
various important surgical processes. Telerobotic systems are used for diagnostic
methods such as USG (ultrasonographic) scanning and biopsy, and also for serious
interventions including surgical processes. Though AESOP was used successfully
during the 1990s, the Zeus robotic system was used for laparoscopy as the first
robotic system for telesurgery in "Operation Lindbergh" in 2001 [24]. Telerobotics
uses the "master–slave" approach to control the robotic system from far away.
MELODY is an established telerobotics system that is being used successfully for
multiple surgeries [25]. The main types of telerobot configurations include both
simple serial and complex parallel robotic systems [26, 27], and specific types such
as snakes [28] and Pop-Up manufacture of microelectromechanical systems
(MEMS). A modern telerobotic system requires appropriate logical network architecture, enhanced connectivity, and an interruption-free network. Special attention
should be given to real-time, high-quality live video streaming, data controlling,
data storage, and information gathering. The present 4G data network connectivity
is serving well; however, the 5G network and increasing implementation of the
Internet of Things (IoT) could change the overall experience [29].

3.4   Application of Internet of Things (IoT) in Robotic Surgery

The increased application of internet-based technologies has allowed huge bodies of data to be exchanged in different forms between two or more connection points. The integrated technologies of the Internet of Things (IoT) have helped to connect multiple embedded systems and exchange crucial information even in a real-time situation. Furthermore, improved connectivity with 5G or beyond will improve such runtime data exchange and allow most tasks to be controlled remotely. Hence, such technological applications are finding excellent applications in distance-based robotic surgery, designated the Internet of Robotic Things (IoRT) [30]. Several recent reports suggest that attempts in this direction have already been initiated. In minimally invasive surgery, IoRT-based HTC VIVE PRO controllers for redundant manipulators were used for smooth human–robot interactions, and better performance was recorded [30]. Ishak and Kit recently reported the application of IoRT in robot-assisted surgeries [31].

3.5   Virtual Reality (VR) and Augmented Reality (AR) in Robotic Surgery

Virtual reality (VR) refers to interaction with a computer simulation-derived and artificially-generated 3D environment. It was initially popular in computer gaming. Soon it was realized that VR could be useful in a serious context such as live surgery monitoring rather than just for entertainment. Such customized simulation system protocols are immensely useful in modern-day critical training that is expensive and risky. Hence, VR-based technologies are being used extensively in simulation exercises for pilots as well as training robotic surgeons. Applications of VR for training laparoscopic surgeons have been reported [32, 33]. Several more recent applications of VR have also been reported for such training, surveyed extensively by Bric et al. and others [34]. Recent advances in specific surgical processes such as vesicourethral anastomosis and improving motor skills are also reported to have used VR-based techniques [35, 36]. Augmented reality (AR)-dependent methods are also being used for training surgeons to improve connections with the real world for a surgical process associated with robot-assisted surgeries such as neurosurgery [37] and others [38].

3.6   Artificial Intelligence (AI) and Deep Learning (DL) in Robotic Surgery

Artificial intelligence (AI) has revolutionized sophisticated modern data analysis methods and made information processing more meaningful and effective. The real-time application of AI is remarkable in almost all fields of science and technology. Broad and specific applications of AI technologies and algorithms such as Artificial Neural Network (ANN) and others have been reported from molecular biology to advanced medicine [39, 40]. AI is being used extensively in medical sciences and allied subjects [41], from the initial conversation with a patient through Chatbots to critical surgical operations. The futuristic telemedicine system is applying AI-derived technologies along with advanced robotics [42]. AI algorithms are now part of medical diagnosis, specifically in disease diagnosis from clinical images [43]; advanced deep learning tools are used to diagnose autism from MRI images [44]. Numerous similar successful applications have proved the efficiency of machine learning (ML) and deep learning (DL) technologies in medical problem-solving and improving diagnosis and patient care system.

4 Levels of Autonomy for Robotic Systems

As time passes, systems dependent on robotics and AI are becoming more reliable and autonomous in many ways. However, strict guidelines on the limit of autonomy are needed for these systems owing to concerns about extensive applications. Human interference is inevitable, and major decisions must be considered by humans. Restricted guidelines have recently been issued by the FDA in response to growing complaints from patients [22]. Nevertheless, specific robotic autonomy is the need of the moment, and it is challenging to design and develop such robots precisely [45]. Hence, complete autonomy is currently impossible. The different robotic systems used for surgeries are currently automated to different extents; for instance, the da Vinci® surgical system is operated under direct control, the ACROBAT system is managed under shared control, and supervised autonomy is followed for the CyberKnife system [46]. Therefore, the precise scope of autonomy should be defined in each case. Maximum automation could be allowed for repetitive and general mechanical tasks, whereas for certain delicate operations decision-making should be supervised by human experts.

5 Future Directions for Neurosurgical Robots

The robot has become an excellent technology for assisting neurological treatments. It is used in diagnosis, surgery, and rehabilitation (Fig. 1). The modern range of robotics has extended greatly from the earlier basic and general applications. Regarding future directions, this review-evidence demonstrates that the advanced tenet concepts and the development of neurosurgical robots had different origins but have progressed in parallel. Because of acceptance-driven developments including (1) advances in medical imaging technology, (2) engineering technological improvements such as control theory, sensors and actuators, (3) IoT and the 5G network, (4) smart materials, and (5) cell-based therapy and OMICS, they have finally joined. In future, they will progress together. Support from robotics-assisted systems has helped to improve patient care, prosthetics, orthotic device functioning, and surgical interventions. The patient's quality of life after surgery depends on neuroplasticity, a slow and steady process with neurorehabilitation. Hence, neurorehabilitation

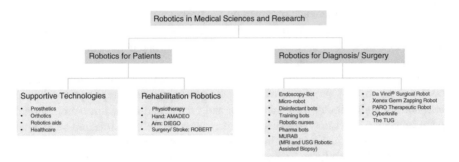

Fig. 1 Presentation of diverse categories of robotics currently implemented in medical sciences

requires constant care and monitoring of patients. These types of robotic assistance that are helping patients to gain normal or improved functionality of their limbs, improving their neuromuscular function, and so on, are enormously beneficial. COBOT, an abbreviation of Collaborative Robot, is specifically designed and programmed to work directly and interact with surgeons within the collaborative workspace. Its advanced features including hand guiding mode, safety monitoring, and power and force limitation represent the future trend for neurosurgical robots.

5.1   Focus on Enhancing the Overall Accuracy and Efficacy of Target Acquisition

5.1.1   Robots for Stereotactic Brain Biopsy and Spinal Surgery

Brain biopsies can be obtained successfully using modern robotic applications. Tissue samples are collected by navigating an advanced robotic system. A recent report by Dlaka and colleagues mentioned that a RONNA G3 robotic system successfully collected brain tissue through a sedan biopsy needle from a patient with B-cell lymphoma [47]. A systematic review Marcus et al. [48] on reports from the last 30 years suggested that stereotactic brain biopsy with robotic assistance is becoming common practice. However, a further detailed evaluation of processes conducted through robotic systems has been recommended for conclusive evidence. A study on 60 patients by Terrier et al. recommended that robot-assisted frameless surgery should be complementary to the frame-based surgical process [49]. The surgical process was safe and surgery time was reduced effectively. Enhanced safety was also noted for a semiautonomous stereotactic brain biopsy [50]. The introduction of novel minimally invasive robotics-based techniques for brain biopsy was feasible for most patients owing to their ease of operation, safety, better accuracy, and efficiency [51]. A similar robot-assisted process by the Neuromate robot (Renishaw, Gloucestershire, UK) was also considered for the brainstem biopsy of children and caused no complications [52]. Comparison of the minimally invasive robot-guided procedure with the manual arm-based protocol corroborated the safety, increased accuracy, and reduced operation time for the robot-assisted technique [53]. The evidence obtained on the growing reliability and safety of the robot-guided technique in operating complex brain biopsy is benefiting patients and surgeons. However, a case-to-case analysis is important and human expertise should not be ignored depending on the circumstances.

Apart from brain biopsy, advanced robotics is being increasingly used for spinal cord surgery. Spinal surgery is tedious and time-consuming, requiring a constant long-term detailed focus with a firm grip and understanding of three-dimensional neuromuscular structures. Advanced robotics with detailed 3D imaging and spinal reconstruction information and fine navigation systems can surely help to replace the required motor skills and repetitive tasks effectively, under careful supervision [54]. Analysis of the growing implementation of robotics applications in spinal surgery suggests that surgical accuracy has improved; nevertheless, the effect of radiation in relation to the robotic surgery type should be studied in detail for spinal surgery [55]. Recently, a real-time image guidance system for robotic assistance was successfully implemented in spinal surgery [56]. It provided better accuracy and improved surgical outcomes, and reduced collateral damage under expert supervision in most cases.

5.1.2   Robots in Intraoperative Imaging (CT/MRI)

Imaging techniques such as computed tomography (CT) scans and magnetic resonance imaging (MRI) are integral to modern pathological diagnosis. These techniques are superior and efficient in most cases. Robot-guided stereoelectroencephalography (sEEG) with 3T MRI conducted on five patients suggested that the process can reduce the radiation exposure of patients and is safe, with improved accuracy in 1.5T MRI [57]. Superior accuracy has been reported for the robotic system associated with tomographical imaging for surgery [58]. Chenin et al. suggested that the Robotic Stereotactic Assistance (ROSA) technique along with flat-panel computed tomography (fpCT) provided higher accuracy in pedicle screwing for circumferential lumbar arthrodesis [59]. Coupling sophisticated imaging techniques with robotics helped to augment accuracy and maintain safety and good patient outcomes. Like CT, MRI has also been coupled with robotics for better results. An integrated system combining MRI and robotics, Stormram 3, has been developed for breast biopsy [60]. Similar MRI and robotics-coupled technology has been developed for neurological rehabilitation [61].

5.1.3   Robotized LASER Ablation

LASER ablation is a minimally invasive procedure for targeted microsurgery of tissues, removed by an iMRI-guided targeted laser. This surgical process has been used frequently for localized tumors such as brain tumors. Currently, ROSA is being used for better targeting and focusing during the ablation process. This technique has been applied to intractable epilepsy [62], necrosis of the posterior cranial fossa [63], and other conditions. Integrated global efforts such as LASER Ablation of Abnormal Neurological Tissue using Robotic NeuroBlate System (LAANTERN) have been developed for better application and analysis of LASER ablation surgery such as brain tumor ablation [64], and safety of Stereotactic LASER ablation (SLA) for intracranial lesions [16]. LASER ablation has emerged as a state-of-the-art procedure for targeted surgical removal of tissues. Further studies and detailed analysis of the results of more cases will provide useful information on the specific success of this technique.

5.2   Focus on Enhancing the Neurosurgeon's Capabilities

5.2.1   Robots for Craniotomy
At present, craniotomy is mostly conducted using semi-automatic tools. The manual process entails many risks including shaking, recoil motion, and others that can affect the outcome of this high-risk procedure. The kinematic process has been optimized and used for robotic applications with better results. Reconfigurable parameters have been studied keenly and a Spherical Parallel Mechanism (SPM) has been proposed for better kinematics during craniotomy through robotic assistance [65]. Development of human–robot interactions and collaborations for craniotomy has been reported [66]. Experiments have been conducted on cadavers to elucidate the kinematics and the force optimization for craniotomy using a long-distance teleoperated robot [65]. Robotics now serves as a regular instrumental process for craniotomy. In the future, with more kinematic studies and optimization, improved automation and skillful implementation will be possible for serious cases.

5.2.2   Robots for Interventional Neurosurgery
Implementation of robotics coupled with interventional MRI was attempted previously [67]. Surgical prototype development and improved accuracy were attempted to achieve better and more reliable implementation of robotics in neurosurgery [68, 69]. Robotics is now regularly used in cerebrovascular and endovascular neurosurgery and is helpful in processes such as intraoperative imaging, catheter introduction and guidance, and navigation [70].

5.2.3   Robots for Endoscopic Endonasal Transsphenoidal Approach
The endoscopic endonasal transsphenoidal approach is a minimally invasive technique for surgical treatment of intrasellar lesions and pituitary adenomas. The transsphenoidal midline-route pathway to reach the intrastellar region offers a sufficient workspace with endoscope-enhanced illumination and panoramic wide-angled view of the supersellar and parasellar portions of intrasellar lesions. When the endoscopic endonasal transsphenoidal approach was first introduced, insertion of an endoscope was a key challenge for neurosurgeons. The development of surgical techniques and improvement of instruments made this approach more promising. Its limitations are surgical difficulties and instrument dexterity. Neurosurgeons have to be tremendously skillful because they operate in a narrow workspace and must be able to reach the exact target, which remains surrounded by eloquent structures including major vascular and neural structures. A human error such as a slight deviation of the tools can lead to undesirable and even fatal consequences. This indicates the requirement for new modalities to assist neurosurgeons. Implementation

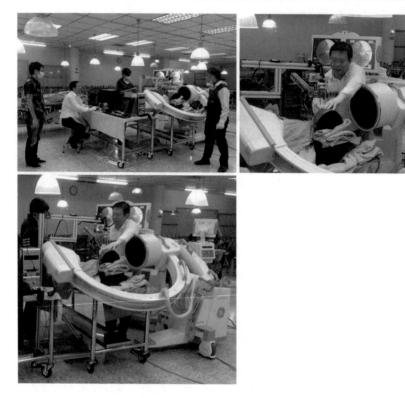

Fig. 2 Presentation of the implementation of robotics for the endoscopic endonasal transsphenoidal approach in a cadaveric study

of robotics for the endoscopic endonasal transsphenoidal approach was attempted in a cadaveric study (Fig. 2). This technology is now considered a crucial modality, with some preclinical research teams working to develop prototype robots. For designing a robot to guide the endoscopic endonasal transsphenoidal approach, the following significant points must be considered: (1) the automation of the task must save time for the neurosurgeon and enhance their competence, (2) the robot must be reliable, i.e. must have in-depth knowledge of the workspace and types of interactions between the instruments it holds and the tissues, and (3) the robot must be very small and easy to install in the operating room, and easily maneuverable by the surgeon [71]. The first cadaveric trial of a robot-guided endoscopic endonasal transsphenoidal approach showed a significantly shorter initial setup process and time of operation than the conventional manual approach [72–75].

5.3   Outlook for the Neurosurgical Robot

The growing application of advanced robotics in neurosurgery and other complex operating procedures provides extensive benefits to patients and neurosurgeons, and helps in reducing procedural complications and probable human errors by focusing on the overall accuracy of neurosurgical procedures and enhancing neurosurgeons' capabilities. However, the improvements are ongoing and require further precise changes in the future. Several significant factors that should be considered are discussed below. First, advanced intraoperative imaging should be included to access, monitor, analyze, and understand real-time data without any interruption or compromised image quality. Image quality and filtering of mechanical shaking in real time are important and can decide the outcome of the neurosurgical process. Second, successful and result-oriented human–machine interface development is essential; proper simulation even with 3D printed models and guided practice should be accessible for training neurosurgeons. Precision can be improved with better 3D image quality, image streaming speed, and processing, minute operating, and distance-based control of the systems during a procedure. Third, the improvement of a parallel network of robotic systems and better data transfer through IoT with the 5G network will yield enormous benefits for operations and neurosurgical work. The autonomy of the robotic systems should be decided after detailed evaluation of individual process and requirements. Further improvement in the autonomy of robotic applications will improve outcomes. Last but not least, reducing the cost of the neurosurgical robot can make the surgeries affordable for most patients. Finally, the effect of the COVID-19 pandemic on surgical practice is a crucial example of its widespread impact on the workforce, staffing issues, procedural prioritization, and interoperative viral transmission risk [76].

Besides the future value of the neurosurgical robot in enhancing the accuracy of neurosurgical procedures and neurosurgeons' capabilities, the effect of the COVID-19 pandemic on neurosurgery is a matter of concern. Most neurosurgical procedures including spine and cranial procedures are safe to perform with strict PPE, but the involvement of neurosurgical robots has to be investigated. PCR testing for COVID-19 is recommended for suspected patients before surgery and the indicated patient should be operated as gently as possible in a negative pressure operating room. To reduce bone aerosol, cranial and spinal drilling should be performed meticulously under robotic assistance. Furthermore, endonasal procedures should be avoided because of significant aerosol droplets and the risk of viral transmission [77, 78].

In this hazardous and uncertain situation, there is a greater role for the robot to enhance health care provider safety, though there are recommendations for prioritization of procedures that involve robotic surgery with the validation guidelines and alterations to operative techniques. To maximize protection for healthcare providers and minimize collateral damage to COVID-19 patients requiring surgery, the robot is needed for procedure-specific reduction of bone aerosol, shortening the time for attaining the target, and distancing the infected patient from the surgical team. Moreover, under robotic-assisted neurosurgery, operations are undertaken only by the most experienced surgeons with the minimum number of staff in the OR. Also, other recommendations need to be followed including (1) adequate use of PPE for all patients, with higher levels of PPE for all healthcare providers, (2) careful selection of patients for all elective surgery, (3) postponement if possible, and (4) minimizing aerosol dispersal.

6   Conclusion

Robotic-assisted neurosurgery has emerged as great support for diagnosis and surgical procedures. It has reduced complex neurosurgical timings and the risk of human error, enhanced the remote control of operation procedures, and increased the affordability and accessibility of a better and more reliable health system. Apart from neurosurgery, robot-assisted systems are being considered for other areas of surgery including gynecological, cardiological, urological, transoral, thoracic, and many more. Enhanced simulation training, and a growing number of professionals with hands-on robot training-assisted neurosurgery, will aid in managing a large pool of patients efficiently and reliably. However, neurosurgical accreditation for robotic procedures is required. Consequently, compliance with standards and ethical considerations such as patient experience, marketing of the robotic surgery systems, cost-effectiveness, the privacy of patient data during remote operations, and responsibility for errors should also be seriously considered.

References

1. Carlsson LMS, Sjöholm K, Jacobson P, Andersson-Assarsson JC, Svensson P-A, Taube M, et al. Life expectancy after bariatric surgery in the Swedish obese subjects study. N Engl J Med. 2020;383(16):1535–43.
2. Cutler DM, Chernow M, Ghosh K, Landrum MB. Understanding the improvement in disability free life expectancy in the U.S. elderly population. In: Insights in the economics of aging. Chicago: University of Chicago Press and The National Bureau of Economic Research; 2017.
3. Mason MT. Creation myths: the beginnings of robotics research. IEEE Robot Automat Mag. 2012;19(2):72–7.
4. Murphy RR. Introduction to AI robotics. The MIT Press; 2019.
5. Ustundag A, Cevikcan E. Industry 4.0: managing the digital transformation; 2017.
6. Dal Mas F, Piccolo D, Cobianchi L, Edvinsson L, Presch G, Massaro M, et al. The effects of artificial intelligence, robotics, and industry 4.0 technologies. Insights from the healthcare sector. In Proceedings of the first European conference on the impact of artificial intelligence and robotics, Oxford; 2019.
7. Faust RA. Robotics in surgery: history, current and future applications. Nova Publishers; 2007.
8. Mittal S, Srinivasan A. Robotics in pediatric urology: evolution and the future. Urol Clin North Am. 2021;48(1):113–25.
9. Mart J-PS, Goh EL, Shah Z. Robotics in total hip arthroplasty: a review of the evolution, application and evidence base. EFORT Open Rev. 2020;5(12):866–73.
10. Qi F, Chen B, She S, S G. Shape sensing and feedback control of the catheter robot for interventional surgery. Indust Robot: Int J Robot Res Appl. 2020.
11. Hu JC, Shoag J. Robotic urology: the next frontier, an issue of urologic clinics. Elsevier; 2020.
12. Asil S, Murat E, Barış VÖ, Görmel S, Çelik M, Yüksel UÇ, et al. Caseous calcification of the mitral annulus; scary image during robotic surgery. J Card Surg. 2020;35(5):1145–7.
13. Kingma BF, Hadzijusufovic E, Van der Sluis PC, Bano E, Lang H, Ruurda JP, et al. A structured training pathway to implement robot-assisted minimally invasive esophagectomy: the learning curve results from a high-volume center. Dis Esophagus. 2020;33(Suppl_2):doaa047.
14. Britz GW, Tomas J, Lumsden A. Feasibility of robotic-assisted neurovascular interventions: initial experience in flow model and porcine model. Neurosurgery. 2020;86(2):309–14.
15. Kumar A, Goyal V, Asaf BB, Trikha A, Sood J, Vijay CL. Robotic thymectomy for myasthenia gravis with or without thymoma-surgical and neurological outcomes. Neurol India. 2017;65(1):58–63.

16. Rennert RC, Khan U, Bartek J, Tatter SB, Field M, Toyota B, et al. Laser ablation of abnormal neurological tissue using robotic neuroblate system (LAANTERN): procedural safety and hospitalization. Neurosurgery. 2020;86(4):538–47.
17. Leal Ghezzi T, Corleta OC. 30 years of robotic surgery. World J Surg. 2016;40(10):2550–7.
18. Shah J, Vyas A, Vyas D. The history of robotics in surgical specialties. Am J Robot Surg. 2014;1(1):12–20.
19. Kwoh YS, Hou J, Jonckheere EA, Hayati S. A robot with improved absolute positioning accuracy for CT guided stereotactic brain surgery. IEEE Trans Biomed Eng. 1988;35(2):153–60.
20. Kazanzides P, Fichtinger G, Hager GD, Okamura AM, Whitcomb LL, Taylor RH. Surgical and interventional robotics - core concepts, technology, and design [tutorial]. IEEE Robot Automat Mag. 2008;15(2):122–30.
21. Lanfranco AR, Castellanos A, Desai JP, Meyers W. Robotic surgery - a current perspective. Ann Surg. 2004;239:14–21.
22. FDA. Computer-assisted surgical systems. Available from: https://www.fda.gov/medical-devices/surgery-devices/computer-assisted-surgical-systems
23. Ramirez PT, Frumovitz M, Pareja R, Lopez A, Vieira M, Ribeiro R, et al. Minimally invasive versus abdominal radical hysterectomy for cervical cancer. N Engl J Med. 2018;379(20):1895–904.
24. Butner SE, Ghodoussi M. Transforming a surgical robot for human telesurgery. IEEE Trans Robot Autom. 2003;19(5):818–24.
25. Vieyres P, Novales C, Rivas R, Vilcahuaman L, Sandoval Arévalo JS, Clark T, et al. The next challenge for WOrld wide Robotized Tele-Echography eXperiment (WORTEX 2012): from engineering success to healthcare delivery; 2013.
26. Anderson PL, Mahoney AW, Webster RJ 3rd. Continuum reconfigurable parallel robots for surgery: shape sensing and state estimation with uncertainty. IEEE Robot Automat Lett. 2017;2(3):1617–24.
27. Nelson C, Larbi MA, Zeghloul S. Multi-robot system optimization based on redundant serial spherical mechanism for robotic minimally invasive surgery. Robotica. 2018;37:1–12.
28. Hopkins J, Spranklin B, Gupta S. A survey of snake-inspired robot designs. Bioinspir Biomim. 2009;4:021001.
29. Avgousti S, Christoforou EG, Panayides AS, Voskarides S, Novales C, Nouaille L, et al. Medical telerobotic systems: current status and future trends. Biomed Eng Online. 2016;15(1):96.
30. Su H, Ovur SE, Li Z, Hu Y, Li J, Knoll A, et al., editors. Internet of Things (IoT)-based collaborative control of a redundant manipulator for teleoperated minimally invasive surgeries. 2020 IEEE international conference on robotics and automation (ICRA); 2020.
31. Ishak MK, Kit NM, editors. Design and implementation of robot assisted surgery based on Internet of Things (IoT). 2017 International conference on advanced computing and applications (ACOMP); 2017.
32. Fiedler MJ, Chen SJ, Judkins TN, Oleynikov D, Stergiou N. Virtual reality for robotic laparoscopic surgical training. Stud Health Technol Inform. 2007;125:127–9.
33. Albani JM, Lee DI. Virtual reality-assisted robotic surgery simulation. J Endourol. 2007;21(3):285–7.
34. Bric JD, Lumbard DC, Frelich MJ, Gould JC. Current state of virtual reality simulation in robotic surgery training: a review. Surg Endosc. 2016;30(6):2169–78.
35. Shim JS, Noh TI, Kim JY, Pyun JH, Cho S, Oh MM, et al. Predictive validation of a robotic virtual reality simulator: the tube 3 module for practicing vesicourethral anastomosis in robot-assisted radical prostatectomy. Urology. 2018;122:32–6.
36. Vasudevan MK, Isaac JHR, Sadanand V, Muniyandi M. Novel virtual reality based training system for fine motor skills: towards developing a robotic surgery training system. The international journal of medical robotics + computer assisted surgery. MRCAS. 2020;16(6):1–14.
37. Madhavan K, Kolcun JPG, Chieng LO, Wang MY. Augmented-reality integrated robotics in neurosurgery: are we there yet? Neurosurg Focus. 2017;42(5):E3.
38. Qian L, Wu JY, DiMaio SP, Navab N, Kazanzides P. A review of augmented reality in robotic-assisted surgery. IEEE Trans Med Robot Bion. 2020;2(1):1–16.

39. Banerjee AK, Ravi V, Murty US, Shanbhag AP, Prasanna VL. Keratin protein property based classification of mammals and non-mammals using machine learning techniques. Comput Biol Med. 2013;43(7):889–99.
40. Bao G, Fang H, Chen L, Wan Y, Xu F, Yang Q, et al. Soft robotics: academic insights and perspectives through bibliometric analysis. Soft Robot. 2018;5(3):229–41.
41. Hamet P, Tremblay J. Artificial intelligence in medicine. Metab Clin Exp. 2017;69s:S36–40.
42. Bhaskar S, Bradley S, Sakhamuri S, Moguilner S, Chattu VK, Pandya S, et al. Designing futuristic telemedicine using artificial intelligence and robotics in the COVID-19 era. Front Public Health. 2020;8(708):556789.
43. Loh E. Medicine and the rise of the robots: a qualitative review of recent advances of artificial intelligence in health. BMJ Leader. 2018;2(2):59–63.
44. Emerson RW, Adams C, Nishino T, Hazlett HC, Wolff JJ, Zwaigenbaum L, et al. Functional neuroimaging of high-risk 6-month-old infants predicts a diagnosis of autism at 24 months of age. Sci Transl Med. 2017;9(393)
45. Thondiyath A. Autonomy for robots: design and developmental challenges (keynote address). Proc Technol. 2016;23:4–6.
46. Yip M, Das N. Robot autonomy for surgery. 2017.
47. Dlaka D, Švaco M, Chudy D, Jerbić B, Šekoranja B, Šuligoj F, et al. Brain biopsy performed with the RONNA G3 system: a case study on using a novel robotic navigation device for stereotactic neurosurgery. The international journal of medical robotics + computer assisted surgery. MRCAS. 2018;14(1)
48. Marcus HJ, Vakharia VN, Ourselin S, Duncan J, Tisdall M, Aquilina K. Robot-assisted stereotactic brain biopsy: systematic review and bibliometric analysis. Childs Nerv Syst. 2018;34(7):1299–309.
49. Terrier L, Gilard V, Marguet F, Fontanilles M, Derrey S. Stereotactic brain biopsy: evaluation of robot-assisted procedure in 60 patients. Acta Neurochir. 2019;161(3):545–52.
50. Minxin Y, Li W, Chan T, Chiu P, Li Z. A semi-autonomous stereotactic brain biopsy robot with enhanced safety. IEEE Robot Automat Lett. 2020;5:1.
51. Minchev G, Kronreif G, Ptacek W, Dorfer C, Micko A, Maschke S, et al. A novel robot-guided minimally invasive technique for brain tumor biopsies. J Neurosurg. 2019;18:1–9.
52. Dawes W, Marcus HJ, Tisdall M, Aquilina K. Robot-assisted stereotactic brainstem biopsy in children: prospective cohort study. J Robot Surg. 2019;13(4):575–9.
53. Minchev G, Kronreif G, Ptacek W, Kettenbach J, Micko A, Wurzer A, et al. Frameless stereotactic brain biopsies: comparison of minimally invasive robot-guided and manual arm-based technique. Operat Neurosurg (Hagerstown, Md). 2020;19:292–301.
54. Overley SC, Cho SK, Mehta AI, Arnold PM. Navigation and robotics in spinal surgery: where are we now? Neurosurgery. 2017;80(3s):S86–s99.
55. Joseph JR, Smith BW, Liu X, Park P. Current applications of robotics in spine surgery: a systematic review of the literature. Neurosurg Focus. 2017;42(5):E2.
56. Ahmed AK, Zygourakis CC, Kalb S, Zhu AM, Molina CA, Jiang B, et al. First spine surgery utilizing real-time image-guided robotic assistance. Comput Assist Surg (Abingdon, Engl). 2019;24(1):13–7.
57. Spyrantis A, Cattani A, Strzelczyk A, Rosenow F, Seifert V, Freiman TM. Robot-guided stereoelectroencephalography without a computed tomography scan for referencing: analysis of accuracy. The international journal of medical robotics + computer assisted surgery. MRCAS. 2018;14(2)
58. Figueroa F, Wakelin E, Twiggs J, Fritsch B. Comparison between navigated reported position and postoperative computed tomography to evaluate accuracy in a robotic navigation system in total knee arthroplasty. Knee. 2019;26(4):869–75.
59. Chenin L, Capel C, Fichten A, Peltier J, Lefranc M. Evaluation of screw placement accuracy in circumferential lumbar arthrodesis using robotic assistance and intraoperative flat-panel computed tomography. World Neurosurg. 2017;105:86–94.
60. Groenhuis V, Veltman J, Siepel F, Stramigioli S. Stormram 3: a magnetic-resonance-imaging-compatible robotic system for breast biopsy. IEEE Robot Automat Magaz. 2017;24(2):34–41.

61. Hong Kai Y, Kamaldin N, Jeong Hoon L, Nasrallah FA, Goh JCH, Chen-Hua Y. A magnetic resonance compatible soft wearable robotic glove for hand rehabilitation and brain imaging. IEEE Trans Neural Syst Rehabil Eng. 2017;25(6):782–93.
62. Gonzalez-Martinez J, Vadera S, Mullin J, Enatsu R, Alexopoulos AV, Patwardhan R, et al. Robot-assisted stereotactic laser ablation in medically intractable epilepsy: operative technique. Neurosurgery. 2014;10(Suppl 2):167–72. discussion 72–3
63. Chan AY, Tran DK, Gill AS, Hsu FP, Vadera S. Stereotactic robot-assisted MRI-guided laser thermal ablation of radiation necrosis in the posterior cranial fossa: technical note. Neurosurg Focus. 2016;41(4):E5.
64. Kim AH, Tatter S, Rao G, Prabhu S, Chen C, Fecci P, et al. Laser ablation of abnormal neurological tissue using robotic NeuroBlate system (LAANTERN): 12-month outcomes and quality of life after brain tumor ablation. Neurosurgery. 2020;87(3):E338–e46.
65. Essomba T, Hsu Y, Sandoval Arévalo JS, Laribi MA, Zeghloul S. Kinematic optimization of a reconfigurable spherical parallel mechanism for robotic assisted craniotomy. J Mech Robot. 2019;11:1.
66. Zhan Y, Duan X, Cui T, Han D, editors. Craniotomy robot system based on human-machine parallel collaboration. In: 2016 IEEE international conference on mechatronics and automation; 2016.
67. Lwu S, Sutherland G. The development of robotics for interventional MRI. Neurosurg Clin Am. 2009;20:193–206.
68. Louw DF, Fielding T, McBeth PB, Gregoris D, Newhook P, Sutherland GR. Surgical robotics: a review and neurosurgical prototype development. Neurosurgery. 2004;54(3):525–36. discussion 36–7
69. Haidegger T, Xia T, Kazanzides P, editors. Accuracy improvement of a neurosurgical robot system 2008. In: 2nd IEEE RAS & EMBS international conference on biomedical robotics and biomechatronics; 2008.
70. Menaker SA, Shah SS, Snelling BM, Sur S, Starke RM, Peterson EC. Current applications and future perspectives of robotics in cerebrovascular and endovascular neurosurgery. J Neurointervent Surg. 2018;10(1):78–82.
71. Trévillot V, Garrel R, Dombre E, Poignet P, Sobral R, Crampette L. Robotic endoscopic sinus and skull base surgery: review of the literature and future prospects. Eur Ann Otorhinolaryngol Head Neck Dis. 2013;130(4):201–7.
72. Chumnanvej S, Chalongwongse S, Pillai BM, Suthakorn J. Pathway and workspace study of Endonasal Endoscopic Transsphenoidal (EET) approach in 80 cadavers. Int J Surg Open. 2019;16:22–8.
73. Chumnanvej S, Madhavan Pillai B, Suthakorn J. Surgical robotic technology for developing an endonasal endoscopic transsphenoidal surgery (EETS) robotic system. The Open Neurol J. 2019;13:96–106.
74. Chumnanvej S, Pattamarakha D, Sudsang T, Suthakorn J. Anatomical workspace study of endonasal endoscopic transsphenoidal approach. Open Med (Wars). 2019;14:537–44.
75. Chumnanvej S, Pillai BM, Chalongwongse S, Suthakorn J. Endonasal endoscopic transsphenoidal approach robot prototype: a cadaveric trial. Asian J Surg. 2020;44(1):345–51.
76. Al-Jabir A, Kerwan A, Nicola M, Alsafi Z, Khan M, Sohrabi C, et al. Impact of the coronavirus (COVID-19) pandemic on surgical practice - part 1. Int J Surg. 2020;79:168–79.
77. Society of British Neurological Surgeons. 2020. Available from: https://www.sbns.org.uk/index.php/download_file/view/1642/416/.
78. British Neuro-Oncology Society. COVID-19 treatment pathways and guidance 2020. Available from: https://www.bnos.org.uk/clinical-practice/treatment-pathways-and-guidance/.

Printed in the United States
by Baker & Taylor Publisher Services